Porcelain & Composite Inlays & Onlays

Esthetic Posterior Restorations

David A. Garber, DMD • **Ronald E. Goldstein, DDS**

Porcelain & Composite Inlays & Onlays

Esthetic Posterior Restorations

David A. Garber, DMD

Clinical Professor of Periodontics
Medical College of Georgia
School of Dentistry
Augusta, Georgia

Clinical Professor of Prosthodontics
Medical College of Georgia
School of Dentistry
Augusta, Georgia

Special Lecturer in Esthetic Dentistry
Emory University
School of Dentistry
Atlanta, Georgia

Private Practice, Atlanta, Georgia

Ronald E. Goldstein, DDS

Clinical Professor
  of Restorative Dentistry
Medical College of Georgia
School of Dentistry
Augusta, Georgia

Special Lecturer in Esthetic Dentistry
Emory University
School of Dentistry
Atlanta, Georgia

Adjunct Clinical Professor
  of Prosthodontics
Boston University
Goldman School of Graduate Dentistry
Boston, Massachusetts

Private Practice, Atlanta, Georgia

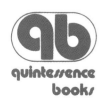

quintessence books

Quintessence Publishing Co, Inc
Chicago, Berlin, London, Tokyo, Moscow, Sofia, and Warsaw

Library of Congress Cataloging-in-Publication Data

Garber, David A.
    Porcelain & composite inlays & onlays: esthetic posterior
restorations / David A. Garber, Ronald E. Goldstein.
       p.   cm.
    Includes bibliographical references and index.
    ISBN 0-86715-171-4
    1. Inlays (Dentistry). 2. Dental ceramics. 3. Dental acid
etching. I. Goldstein, Ronald E. II. Title. III. Title:
Porcelain and composite inlays and onlays.
    [DNLM: 1. Dental Porcelain. 2. Inlays. 3. Acid Etching, Dental.
WU 360 G213e 1993]
    RK519.P65G37   1994
    617.6'75—dc20
    DNLM/DLC
    for Library of Congress   93-19866
                                                CIP

quintessence
books

Composition: Focus Graphics, St Louis, MO
Printing and Binding: Everbest Printing Co, Ltd, Hong Kong
Printed in Hong Kong

Contents

To Dr Ralph Phillips, professor of dental
material science—friend and mentor to us all,
who gave generously of his time, talent,
and wonderful sense of humor.

Contributors

Pinhas Adar, CDT
Master Ceramist
Adar Laboratories, Atlanta, Georgia

Barry P. Isenberg, DMD, MA
Professor
Fixed Prosthodontics Section
Department of Restorative Dentistry
University of Alabama
School of Dentistry
Birmingham, Alabama

Karl F. Leinfelder, DDS, MS
Alumni/Volker Professor of
   Clinical Dentistry,
Director of Biomaterials Clinical Research,
   and Acting Chairman
Department of Biomaterials
University of Alabama
School of Dentistry
Birmingham, Alabama

Leonard Litkowski, DDS, MS
Assistant Professor
Program in Dental Materials
Department of General Dentistry
University of Maryland
Baltimore College of Dental Surgery
Baltimore, Maryland

Dan Nathanson, DMD, MSD
Professor and Chairman
Department of Biomaterials
Director, Division of Continuing Education
Boston University
Goldman School of Graduate Dentistry
Boston, Massachusetts

Howard Strassler, DMD, FADM
Associate Professor and Director of
   Operative Dentistry
Department of General Dentistry
University of Maryland
Baltimore College of Dental Surgery
Baltimore, Maryland

Preface

This book is about choices — alternatives to conventional posterior amalgam restorations. The evolution of dental materials has provided dentistry with a variety of solutions to the problem of carious or discolored posterior teeth. For centuries now, dental amalgam has been the general standard by which dentists and materials have been measured. In recent years the practice of routinely restoring teeth with amalgam has again been questioned, but, regardless of any controversy about the possible effects of mercury, today we can offer our patients choices to consider when we restore their posterior teeth. This book therefore provides possible solutions for the millions of people who would like an answer to the question, "Are there any alternatives?"

The concept of using porcelain as an intracoronal restoration is not really new, but in the past such restorations were not particularly successful, predominantly because of the lack of an effective cementation medium. The ability to etch porcelain with hydrofluoric acid (as is used for porcelain laminate veneers), coupled with the dual-bonding effect of composite resin to enamel and dentin, has made this intracoronal restoration and the heat-cured indirect composite resin restoration definitive options, especially compared to the compromises faced with amalgam, gold, direct composite resin restorations, and full-coverage restorations.

This text is a procedural atlas on the state of the art of this exciting new technique. It also offers a look at the future trends involving CAD/CAM and other computer modalities.

Acknowledgments

Any book represents the endeavors of many different people, and this text is no exception. The manuscript has been typed, retyped, and edited by Candace Paetzhold; Margie Smith, as always, has been there to type, collate, and organize the various aspects of preparing this book for the publisher. Our technicians, Pinhas Adar and Mark Hamilton, together with Larry Lindke, have gone through innumerable different materials, products, and ceramics in trying to develop the most effective solutions to the problems we encountered in refining this relatively new technique. Mr Adar's unique artistry and skills are evident throughout this book. In Switzerland, Dr Peter Schärer and Arnold Wohlwend introduced us to notable new concepts and graciously lent us slides; similarly did Dr Stefan Eidenbenz give us his support. Our staff in general, but in particular Debby Michalec, with the help of Kim Nimmons, spent many late evenings cataloging slide material, research data, and information imperative for this book. Our two partners, Cathy Goldstein Schwartz and Cary Goldstein, have been sources of advice and guidance and have proofread this manuscript whenever necessary.

We would like to acknowledge the technical photographic advice and help received from Mr Howard Golden and Mr John Johnny of the Minolta Corporation. The photographs and slides were all made using the Minolta 7000 with a 100-mm macro lens and the 1200 AF electronic flash unit.

The time needed to write any book has to be taken from somewhere, and this was gleaned from time that should have been spent with our families, in particular our children — Karen, Jennifer, and Michael, and Ken and Rick — as well as our wives, Barbara and Judy. We certainly appreciate their understanding in allowing us to complete this endeavor.

Historical Perspective and Comparison of Posterior Restorations

1

Karl F. Leinfelder

For centuries dentists have tended to divide treatment into anterior and posterior restorations. For a multitude of reasons, anterior teeth have received most of the attention and even a consensus of potential solutions. However, the opposite is true when it comes to posterior teeth. The controversy arises as to the best approach to satisfy patients' esthetic and functional needs to keep their dentitions in optimal condition. Much of the controversy centers on which material best restores posterior teeth. Although amalgam has been universally accepted, the dental profession has also used other materials: gold alloys, composite resins, and various types of ceramic compositions. This chapter briefly discusses these materials.

Amalgam

Dental amalgam has played a key role as a posterior restorative material during the last century.

Although other materials have been developed for the restoration of occlusal surfaces, this early-developed material continues to be the most frequently used.

Its continued popularity is most evident by the fact that it accounts for nearly 75% of all materials used by dentists.

The reasons for the continued acceptance of amalgam are numerous. Compared to other restorative materials, it is relatively simple to use, low in cost, clinically durable, and, perhaps most importantly, it is fairly tolerant of manipulative variation.

The first amalgams used by dentists more than a century ago consisted of coin silver and mercury. While the physical and mechanical characteristics of these amalgams were far from ideal, the concept of inserting a plastic or workable mass into a prepared cavity and then carving it to the desired anatomic form appealed immediately to a large number of clinicians. Such a technique was far faster and more simple than the only alternative, which was condensing pellets of gold foil. Unfortunately, the composition of the early alloys available for generating amalgam restorations differed greatly from one material to another. Similarly, the handling characteristics and general clinical behavior varied appreciably.

Due to the efforts of Black (1896) and Gray (1923), however, the composition of the alloy was dramatically improved. Then in 1929, a standard for amalgam was adopted by the American Dental Association. In effect, it established a range of compositional elements, as well as rigid limits for dimensional changes during amalgamation. Because of these efforts, the profession for the first time was assured that the material being used complied to a standard of acceptability.

Composition

Although the composition of current-day formulations varies, amalgam alloy generally contains more silver than it does any other component. The second most common element is tin, followed by copper. Although zinc may be in the composition, many of the current-day formulations are free of this element. The silver-tin-copper alloy is triturated with pure mercury at a ratio of approximately 1:1.

Nearly 20 years ago, a new type of amalgam alloy was introduced to the profession. Identified as a high-copper–containing amalgam, this innovative material contained copper contents ranging upward from 13%. Some of the more recent formulations contain copper in amounts of nearly 30%. The results of several well-designed clinical studies, it was showed that the new alloys were significantly superior to their low-copper–containing counterparts. The improvement in clinical behavior was shown to be related to the elevated copper content. In principle, the excess copper tends to combine with the tin, thereby reducing or preventing formation of the tin-mercury phase. In the absence of the corrosion-prone gamma II component, the amalgam is considerably more resistant to degradation.

The longevity of high-copper amalgam is normally greater that that of the traditional or low-copper–containing compositions. Specifically, the extent of marginal fracture or ditching is appreciably less. Furthermore, the high-copper amalgams exhibit less surface pitting, volumetric expansion, and flow or creep from the cavity preparation. Finally, this class of materials is even more tolerant of manipulative errors than are conventional compositions.

An example of differences in the clinical performance of conventional and high-copper amalgams is illustrated in Fig 1-1. Shown are two amalgam restorations inserted at the same time. The restoration placed in tooth 14 is Velvalloy (SS White), a conventional composition. The restoration in tooth 15 is a high-copper amalgam, Dispersalloy (Johnson & Johnson). The age of these two restorations is 4 years. Note the apparent differences in the clinical performances of the two restorations. The high-copper amalgam restoration continues to exhibit excellent marginal integrity, whereas the conventional composition is beginning to show strong evidence of marginal deterioration. The same two restorations after 8 years of clinical service are shown in Fig 1-2. The differences in clinical performances of the two restorations are even more appreciable. At this stage the surface of the conventional composition is beginning to break down, whereas the high-copper amalgam restoration continues to exhibit the same type of clinical characteristics that it did at the end of 3 years. The two restorations at the end of 10 years are illustrated in Fig 1-3. Note the severe marginal breakdown of the conventional composition, as well as evidences of flow or creep, not only on the occlusal surface, but also into the interproximal region. By comparison, the high-copper amalgam restoration continues to exhibit excellent clinical characteristics. The same two restorations after 16 years of service are shown in Fig 1-4.

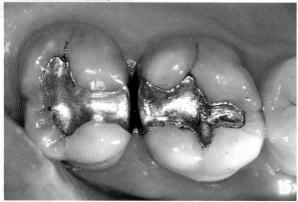

Fig 1–1 Two amalgam restorations, each placed 4 years previously. The restoration on the left is a high-copper amalgam (Dispersalloy) and the one on the right is a conventional amalgam (Velvalloy).

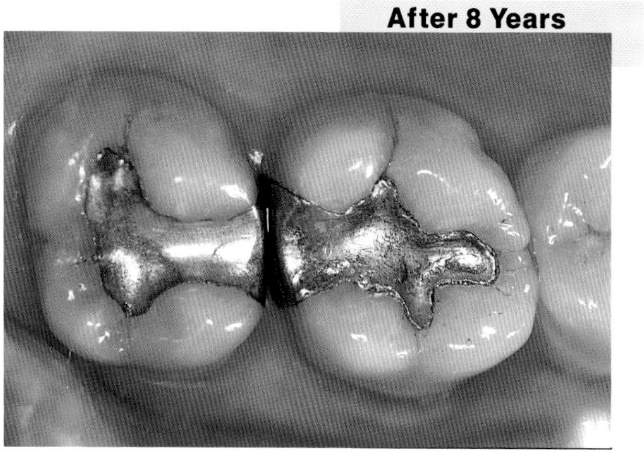

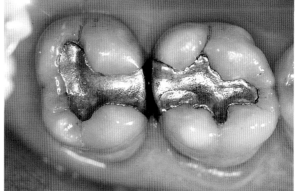

Fig 1–2 Same restorations after 8 years of service.

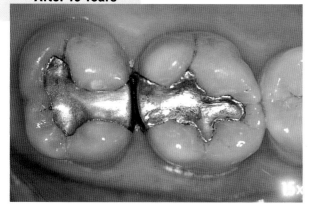

Fig 1–3 Same restorations at the end of 10 years.

Fig 1–4 Same restorations at the end of 16 years.

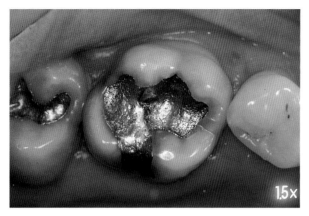

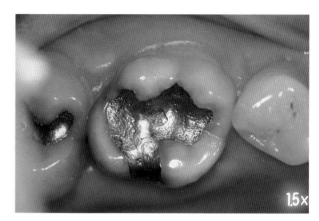

Fig 1–5 Conventional low-copper amalgam restoration has been precarved burnished but not polished, shown 2 years after placement.

Fig 1–6 Same restoration after 3 years.

It should be noted that the amount of residual mercury in the completed restoration plays a major role in the overall corrosion resistance of the restoration. Therefore, clinicians should use whatever technique is effective in reducing excess mercury from the restoration. This effect can be achieved by using the appropriate condensation techniques or with precarve burnishing. Both of these procedures bring the excess mercury to the surface of the restoration, which is then readily removed during the carving process.

The precarve-burnishing technique is so effective that it can actually enhance the clinical performance of a conventional amalgam to the status of the high-copper amalgam. A typical example is illustrated in Figs 1-5 and 1-6.

Figure 1-5 shows a conventional low-copper amalgam restoration that has been precarved burnished but not polished. The age of the restoration is 2 years. The same restoration after 3 years of service is shown in Fig 1-6. Note that there is relatively little difference in marginal integrity despite the age of the restoration.

Amalgam

Advantages

- Material of choice as a direct restorative material for posterior teeth
- Relatively simple to use
- Comparatively unaffected by routine manipulation
- Higher clinical longevity than most other direct restorative materials
- Considerably less expensive than any of its counterparts

Disadvantages

- Considered unesthetic by most patients
- Does not bond the remaining tooth structure together, unlike acid etched and bonded composite resin
- Still unanswered question of dimensional change of amalgam and its possible relation to microcracks
- Corrosive breakdown of older amalgam restorations may cause a structural problem in the form of potential tooth fracture
- Continuing controversy over possible mercury toxicity and antibiotic inhibition

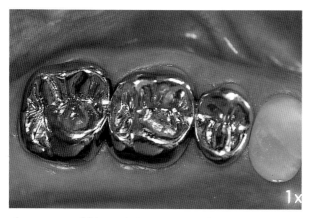

Fig 1–7 Gold-based alloy after several years of clinical service.

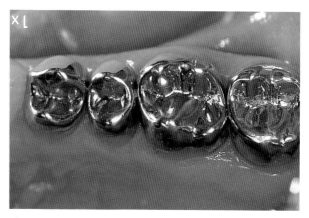

Fig 1–8 Low-gold alloy exhibits excellent tarnish resistance and marginal integrity.

Gold Alloys

Gold-based alloys have long been considered the most ideal material for the restoration of posterior teeth. This type of indirect restorative material can commonly last for 25 to 40 years in the mouths of caries-free patients. Its success is related to a number of factors, including corrosion resistance, relative ease of handling, and excellent physical and mechanical characteristics.

The basic disadvantages of the material are its color, relatively high cost to the patient, and some degree of technique-sensitivity, both clinically and in the laboratory. The use of gold-based alloys for restoring posterior teeth became more common with the development of the lost-wax process early in the 20th century. Improvements in the investment material associated with the casting process in the 1930s made the procedure more predictable, further encouraging the clinician to use this most effective material. Examples of restorations made with gold-based alloys are given in Figs 1-7 and 1-8. Figure 1-9 shows an example of the potential for optimal gap dimension.

Composition

The original gold alloys used by the dental profession were basically coin alloys and consisted of gold, copper, and silver. As time progressed,

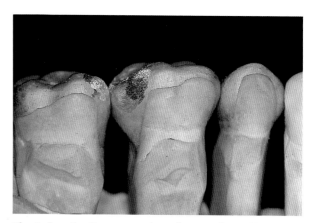

Fig 1–9 Castings seated on die reveal excellent marginal integrity.

the compositions were modified. At present, four basic types of alloys are available to the dental profession. These different groups of alloys have a range of composition and mechanical properties (Tables 1-1 and 1-2).

In recent years a new group of alloys has been introduced to the dental profession. Identified as *low-gold casting alloys*, these new systems essentially contain lower gold content but higher amounts of palladium. The range of gold content for these new alloys varies from approximately 40% to 60%. Palladium contents are as high as 9%. A number of corrosion studies showed

Table 1–1 *Composition of Casting Gold Alloys*

	Au	Ag	Cu	Pt	Pd	Zn
Type 1	85	10	5	0	0	6
Type 2	75	13	8	1	2	1
Type 3	70	15	10	2	2	1
Type 4	65	12	15	3	2	3

Table 1–2 *Average Properties of Gold Alloys*

	VHN	Propositional limit (MPa)	Tensile (MPa)
Type 1	82	85	280
Type 2	105	160	350
Type 3*	120–170	175–300	360–480
Type 4*	175–250	290–550	450–700

*Value depends on method of heat treatments.

that an increased palladium content would compensate for a significant reduction in gold (Gettleman, 1980; Leinfelder et al, 1981). Interestingly, a number of well-controlled clinical studies demonstrated that the low-gold alloys performed equally as well as those of the traditional composition. In general, however, because of the elevated amounts of palladium, most of these systems exhibited higher hardness values. Most of the low-gold alloys were comparable to the Type III gold alloys. The only negative aspect of the low-gold alloy compositions related to their fabrication. As a rule, they were somewhat more technique-sensitive in terms of heating and casting. Prolonged heating caused by improperly regulated torch flames tended to burn off the base metals in the alloy, resulting in pitting and subsequent discoloration within the oral cavity. Interestingly, however, no differences were shown to exist in the precision of the casting fit, castability, or finishing.

Posterior Composite Resins

Composite resins were developed by Bowen (1962) in the early 1960s and were subsequently introduced to the dental profession several years later. Consisting of tough, wear-resistant resin (bis-GMA) and a ceramic filler, this new type of material was superior to earlier tooth-colored restorations in terms of physical and mechanical properties as well as ease of manipulation. After a number of minor modifications, composite resin was recommended for use as a substitute for amalgam in posterior teeth. While initially these restorations looked most favorable when used as occlusal surfaces, long-term clinical studies indicated that the material was, in fact, unacceptable for this purpose. In addition to wearing at a rate of approximately 100 to 150 μm per year (Leinfelder and Roberson, 1983), many of the restored teeth exhibited evidence of secondary caries.

Several years later the 3M Company introduced a modified material recommended for use in posterior restorations. The modification essentially consisted of reducing the mean particle size from approximately 35 to 3 μm and increasing the total filler content from 75 to 86 wt%. Subsequent clinical studies demonstrated that this modification to the filler content resulted in a significant decrease in wear (Leinfelder and Taylor, 1978). When tested under the same conditions, the wear rate was shown to be less than 50 μm per year.

Today these early materials have been considerably improved. A number of commercially available composite resin materials now exhibit wear rates of less than 10 μm per year (Gerbo et al, 1990).

At present, a great variety of composite resins is available to the profession. Although attempts have been made to classify these materials according to particle size, most classification systems are still somewhat confusing. To alleviate this, a simple classification has been suggested (Table 1-3). The basic advantages to this type of a classification are that it is simple, easy, and convenient to use. Each group of composite resins contains filler particles that are smaller or larger than those in the adjacent group by a factor of

Table 1–3 *Classification of Composite Resins According to Size of Filler Particles*

Type	Particle size (μm)	Example	Manufacturer
Conventional	50	Concise	3M Dental
		Adaptic	Johnson & Johnson
Intermediate	1–5	P-50	3M Dental
		Visiomolar RO	ESPE
Fine	0.5–0.9	Herculite XR	Kerr/Sybron
		Charisma	Kulzer
		TPH	Caulk
Microfill	0.05	Helimolar RO	Ivoclar
		Durafill	Kulzer
		Silux Plus	3M Dental

10. Most composite resins for posterior teeth currently contain filler particles belonging to the intermediate group. In other words, most of these materials contain an average particle size of 1 to 5 μm.

There is still another classification of materials, which can be referred to as *hybrid*. Essentially a hybrid is a composite resin containing filler particles of two different sizes. One of the component fillers is a microfill, and the other is of substantially large particle size. All composite resins now on the market contain some microfill component, which makes the use of the term *hybrid* seem somewhat confusing. Small amounts of microfill are commonly added to enhance the handling characteristics, such as packability and resistance to flow. A true hybrid, however, is considered to be a material in which at least 20% to 25% of the total filler content is a microfill, which effectively increases the percentage of filler as determined by volume.

It is desirable to use a composite resin containing about 70% filler by volume.

Today most of the composite resins on the market fall into two major groups: *(1)* those that contain filler particles averaging 1 to 5 μm and *(2)* those in which the majority of the filler content is in the microfill range of around 0.04 μm. The advantage of the latter type of microfill composite resin is that it can be polished to a high degree of surface reflectivity. On the other hand, it has a lower filler content and as a result its strength, flexural fatigue, and modulus of elasticity are somewhat lower. When compared to resins containing a larger filler size, the microfills are more prone to marginal fracture or degradation, localized wear, and bulk fracture; however, their resistance to generalized loss of material is usually superior to those containing larger filler particles.

Considerable progress has been made in developing composite resins that are substantially more wear-resistant than their predecessors, but they still remain one of the most technique-sensitive materials used in dentistry today. Posterior composite resin restorations are considerably more difficult to place and are much more sensitive to variations in technique than are amalgam restorations. Consequently, unless extreme care is used when these restorative agents are inserted, secondary caries can be a very serious problem. The occurrence of secondary caries in association with posterior composite resins is greater than it is with an amalgam restorative material. In addition, secondary caries progresses at a much slower rate in conjunction with amalgam than it does with posterior composite resins.

While secondary caries may sometimes exist underneath the amalgam restoration for 1 year or more, the same is not true for posterior composite resins. Once the secondary caries process is initiated, it may be only a matter of months before it progresses sufficiently to reach the pulp chamber. Although the reason for the differences in the caries rate associated with materials is not totally understood, it appears to be related to the individual chemistry of the two systems. The silver, copper, tin, or even mercury in the amalgam tends to have a bacteriostatic effect. The posterior composite resin has nothing in its component parts to discourage the carious process. This is accompanied by the relatively high differential in coefficient of thermal expansion and the resultant potential for open margins in composite resin restorations; hence the carious process is actively encouraged.

Although composite resins have improved substantially, they cannot yet be considered as substitutes for amalgam any more than amalgam can be considered a substitute for cast restorative materials. Undoubtedly, the posterior composite resins will improve both in wear-resistance and technique-sensitivity as composite resin systems that do not exhibit polymerization shrinkage and can be predictably bonded directly to dentinal surfaces are developed. In the interim, posterior composite resins should only be used selectively and, as a general rule, they should not be used in centric holding areas.

Posterior Composite Resins

Advantages

- Excellent potential for color matching.
- Freedom from possible mercury toxicity.
- Ability to bond to tooth structure.
- Current formulations possess excellent ratios of opacity and translucency, which commonly make it difficult to discern the restorative material from the surrounding tooth structure.
- Increasing strengths of the bond between tooth structure (dentin and enamel) permit the dentist an excellent opportunity for reinforcing the restored tooth rather than simply replacing tooth structure.

Disadvantages

- More technique-sensitive than amalgam—contacts, occlusion, and marginal seal are all difficult to accomplish.
- Require considerably longer periods of time to place successfully than a corresponding amalgam restoration, because of the additional steps and exacting procedures.
- Secondary caries is more prevalent with posterior restorations, progressing more rapidly once established.

Heat-Cured Resin Inlays/Onlays

It is generally agreed that posterior composite resins should not be considered as substitutes for amalgams. As already stated, composite resins do not offer sufficient wear-resistance, they are technique-sensitive, and they are frequently characterized by problems of marginal adaptation. This often leads to the development of secondary caries and problems with tight proximal contacts and proximal contours. With this in mind, the heat-treated composite resin inlay/onlay concept was developed. The introduction was stimulated by the investigations of Wendt (1987), who demonstrated in his in vitro studies that heat treating at 250°F for 7 to 8 minutes substantially improved hardness and wear-resistance of the resins. The procedure is used to generate a conventional inlay or onlay cavity preparation but without occlusal beveling of the cavosurface angle. A separating agent is applied to the walls of the preparation, and the tooth is restored with a composite resin, which is photocured and then removed from the preparation. The restoration is heat treated extraorally for 7 to 8 minutes at 250°F and cemented back into the cavity with a composite resin luting medium. The clinician also has the option of doing this indirectly by taking an impression, thus generating a cast with a die of the prepared tooth. After final contouring and heat-treating, the restoration is cemented into the prepared tooth with a dual-curing composite resin luting agent.

Heat-Cured Resin Inlays/Onlays

Advantages

- Operator has considerably better control over proximal contour and contact and marginal adaptation.
- Compared to conventional composite resin placement, the inlay/onlay systems should provide superior resistance to microleakage and secondary caries. The potential for increased wear-resistance, however, has yet to be determined clinically.

  Research still shows some controversy concerning these products. For instance, in a recent study by Peutzfeldt and Asmussen (1990), the mechanical properties of the indirect composite resin inlay were not improved over those of the conventional restorative composite resin.

Disadvantages

- The composite resin inlay, whether constructed directly or indirectly, requires additional time and skill as compared to direct insertion procedures.
- The inlay or onlay procedure is more expensive for the patient than are conventional direct posterior composite resin placement techniques, because of the increased time required as well as the additional instrumentation. (See chapter 9 for complete clinical details on the technique.)

Features of Etched Porcelain Inlays and Onlays

2

The quest for an esthetic posterior restoration that is both conservative and predictable has plagued the dental profession for many years. Recently the combination of several different facets of operative dentistry has resulted in a most effective solution: *the etched porcelain restoration.*

The concept of a ceramic inlay dates back to the end of the last century, when the first restorations of this type were fabricated. The problems inherent with porcelain, such as material weakness and marginal integrity, combined with the lack of an adequate cementing medium, initially made this an unsuccessful restoration. The recent development of reinforcing systems for porcelain, however, coupled with the ability to etch and bond the porcelain to the underlying etched tooth structure, has allowed these types of restoration to become a part of our day-to-day operative armamentarium. The strength of the restorative material is developed much as brittle enamel is supported on the dentinal core

of the tooth. The enamel is bonded at the dentinoenamel junction to this underlying core of dentin, so that forces placed on any single aspect are dissipated via this junction to the underlying support system — the dentin. The dentin is less calcified and more malleable and therefore tends to effectively distribute and absorb the forces applied to the enamel surface. The advent of stronger, more predictable dentin bonding agents allows us to use this feature so that the core of dentin supports the bonded porcelain, as opposed to the enamel.

Recent research has demonstrated that compromised teeth restored with this type of resin-bonded etched porcelain restoration developed cuspal stiffness and strength equal to, and in some cases exceeding, that of totally unrestored teeth.

These teeth, like other forms of bonded composite resin restorations, developed increased resistance to fracture and increased cuspal stiffness but with simultaneous reduced microleakage.

Indications

The etched porcelain inlay offers three distinct advantages over comparable restorations: *it is more esthetic, it restores strength to compromised teeth, and it is highly conservative.* Hence, any clinical situations involving the following features may benefit from the etched porcelain inlay:

- **Small to moderate carious lesions** (Figs 2–1a to d). The etched porcelain inlay is indicated in those situations where, although restoration strength is not a preeminent factor because of the size of the lesion, the patient still requests a highly esthetic restoration. (Compound cavities should have a thickness of about 2 mm. If less, a composite resin restoration may be preferable.)

- **Large carious or traumatic lesions with undermined enamel to the extent that a cast-metal restoration or a full crown normally becomes necessary** (Figs 2–2a to d). In these situations the cross-linked resin-bonded porcelain restoration will bond to the remaining tooth structure, binding it together in a homogenous mass.

- **The endodontically compromised tooth where the access cavity has compromised the strength and prognosis of the tooth** (Figs 2–3a to d). In many of these situations the only alternative restoration is some form of post-and-core system and a full-coverage crown, the preparation for which would then remove the little remaining tooth substance. The etched porcelain restoration offers a conservative alternative, whereby most of the remaining tooth is retained, restored, and strengthened.

- **Where metal allergy is a factor.** An alternative modality of therapy is necessary, therefore the bonded ceramic restorations are useful.

- **The restoration of teeth in an arch opposed by already present porcelain restorations.** Because porcelain restorations tend to aggressively wear both normal tooth substance and any other form of restoration, an etched porcelain inlay is indicated.

- **Teeth where it is difficult to develop retention form** (Figs 2–4a to d). These may often be restored by using the adhesive nature of the bonded restoration, as opposed to more aggressive means of developing retention, such as periodontal surgical crown lengthening or elective endodontic therapy to develop post retention.

Contraindications

The greatest contraindications to etched porcelain inlays may well be evidence of parafunctional habits and aggressive wear of the dentition.

In addition, although technique-sensitivity in itself is not a contraindication, the problems of maintaining a dry field and obtaining precisely fabricated restorations, with attention to detail in placement, can make this a contraindication in reality.

Small to Moderate Carious
Lesions (Figs 2–1a to d)

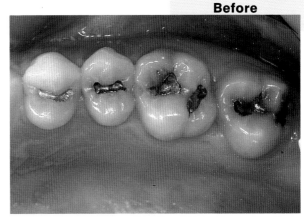

Fig 2–1a Preoperative view of the maxillary left posterior quadrant showing multiple occlusal amalgam restorations in a young patient. Notice the staining associated with caries and the amalgam itself. These types of small restoration might well have been avoided with sealants or preventive resin restorations.

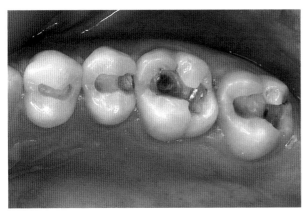

Fig 2–1b Occlusal cavities after removal of the amalgam.

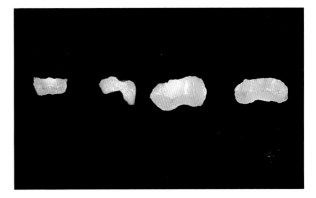

Fig 2–1c Four etched porcelain restorations prior to placement.

After

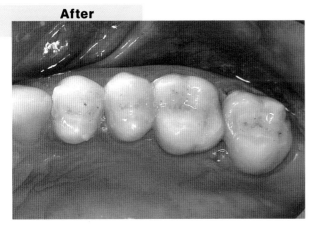

Fig 2–1d Restorations bonded in place. Notice restoration of color, form, and function, with the concomitant strengthening of the teeth.

Large Carious or Traumatic
Lesions (Figs 2–2a to d)

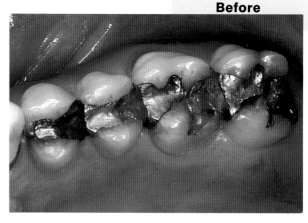

Fig 2–2a   Maxillary left posterior quadrant showing extensive amalgam compound restorations with secondary caries and unsupported tooth structure.

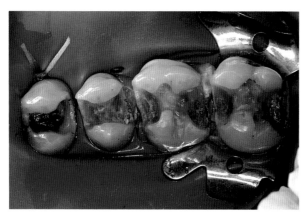

Fig 2–2b   Remaining tooth structure after removal of the amalgam restorations. Notice the wide buccolingual width of the cavities, which usually necessitates onlay preparations and cast-metal restorations to provide strength on the supporting cusps.

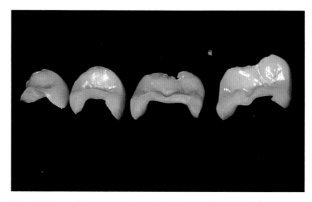

Fig 2–2c   Compound etched porcelain inlays.

After

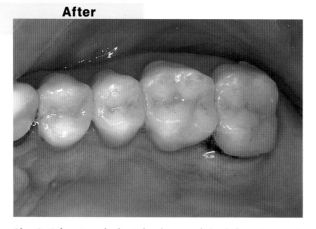

Fig 2–2d   Bonded etched porcelain inlays in position. Notice the restoration of color, form, and function to these highly compromised teeth.

The Endodontically Compromised
Tooth (Figs 2–3a to d)

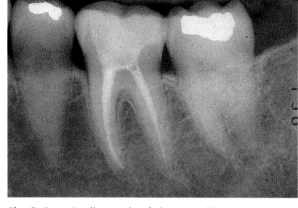

Fig 2–3a Radiograph of the mandibular right first molar after completion of endodontics.

Preparation

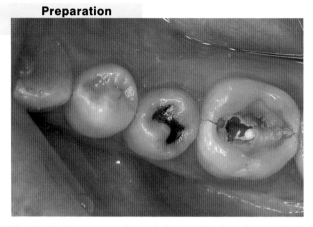

Fig 2–3b Preparation of the molar for the etched, bonded restoration to support the remaining cusps. Notice the endodontic access as well as a mesiodistal fracture. In previous years some form of onlay or full-coverage restoration would usually have been the restoration of choice. With the bonded restoration, cuspal stiffness can be restored without the need for extensive tooth preparations.

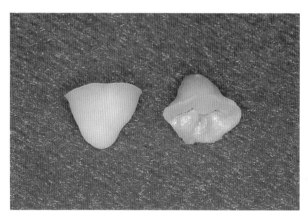

Fig 2–3c Etched restorations before bonding or luting. Note depth of inlay to provide for support through endodontic access. Also note translucency at margins.

After

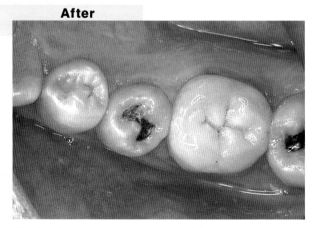

Fig 2–3d Postoperative view of the completed, conservatively restored, but reinforced tooth.

Difficult to Develop Retention
Form (Figs 2–4a to d)

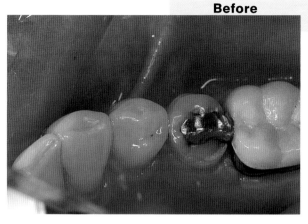

Fig 2–4a Mandibular premolar showing complete fracture of the lingual cusp and remaining amalgam restoration. This type of compromised tooth usually requires a full-coverage restoration.

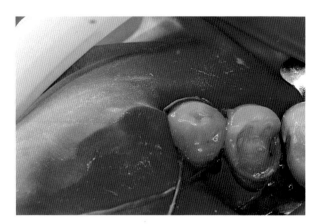

Fig 2–4b The preparation retains all of the remaining tooth structure and does not involve the buccal or mesial aspects of the tooth.

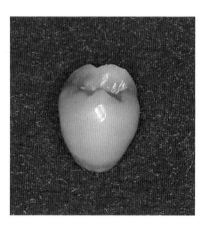

Fig 2–4c The etched porcelain restoration, comprising an occlusal, a lingual, and a distal surface. No retention form is developed for this tooth, merely a resistance form.

After

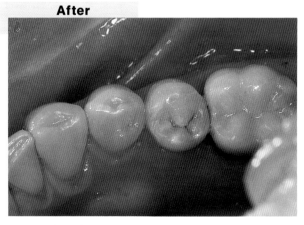

Fig 2–4d The etched porcelain restoration luted in position. Note blend in color to the remaining tooth structure and complete restoration of form and function to this tooth.

Advantages

Porcelain is an excellent replacement material for unesthetic tooth substance (Figs 2–5a to d) for some of the following reasons:

- **Color.** Most porcelain systems use well-established techniques of effectively blending in with the adjacent natural dentition.
- **Periodontal health.** A porcelain restoration may accumulate less plaque on its surface than will other systems.
- **Resistance to abrasion.** The wear- and abrasion-resistance of these restorations is high, although they have the potential to create wear in the opposing arch (Figs 2–6a to c).
- **Radiodensity.** On radiographs, the radiodensity of porcelain resembles that of normal tooth structure, quite often allowing for radiographic access to areas that were previously shielded by radiopaque restorations (Fig 2–7).

Ceramic restorations provide ongoing color, stability, and stain resistance. The marginal integrity, when ceramic restorations are combined with resin bonding and a composite resin luting agent, is excellent with the result that microleakage is decreased to an absolute minimum (Fig 2–8).

Disadvantages

- The amount of time and attention to detail required when these restorations are fabricated and placed (ie, technique-sensitivity) makes them of necessity an expensive alternative to other modalities. Moisture contamination and placement procedures are all potentially problematic.
- The strength of the individual unbonded restoration is relatively nominal, so that the try-in procedures can result in fracture of the porcelain.
- The laboratory fee for this type of restoration is an added factor when a treatment plan is developed.
- The potential for wear of the teeth in the opposing arch, particularly during parafunctional habits, is a contraindication.
- In cast-glass or ceramic restorations with superficial surface stain, occlusal adjustment results in the loss of the surface colorants. This obviously results in a less attractive restoration, when esthetics may well have been the reason the patient sought treatment in the first place.
- Marginal integrity with stacked ceramic may exceed clinically acceptable standards in the case of porcelain onlays.

Conclusion

With the ever-increasing patient awareness and desire for esthetic restorations extending to the posterior regions of the mouth, the new, combined treatment alternative of the etched porcelain resin-bonded restoration is most effective. The only comparable conservative treatment is the posterior composite resin restoration, with the inherent drawbacks of microleakage, polymerization shrinkage, thermal cycling problems, and wear in stress-bearing areas. The bonded restoration has the potential to restore not only esthetics but also strength to previously compromised teeth.

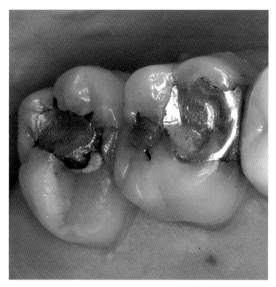

Fig 2–5a Preoperative view of compromised tooth with failing amalgam restoration, fractured cusps, and stained dentin.

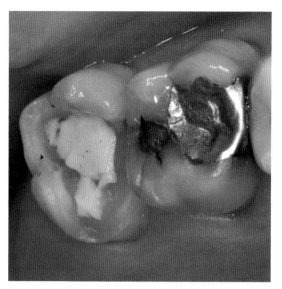

Fig 2–5b Final preparation with base in position, showing missing fractured cusps.

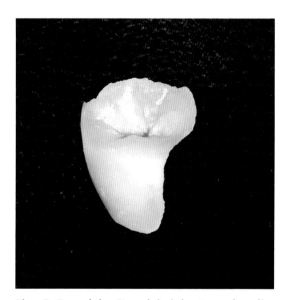

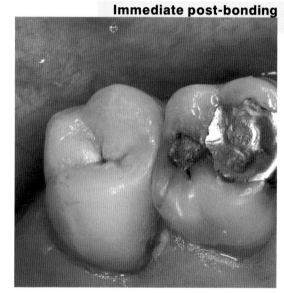

Immediate post-bonding

Figs 2–5c and d Porcelain inlay to replace lingual and occlusal aspects of tooth.

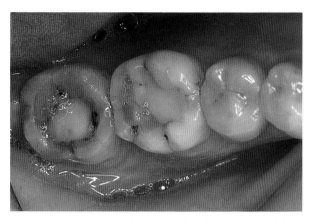

Fig 2–6a Preoperative view showing repeated failure of different restorations on mandibular molar, caused by patient's bruxing habits and opposing ceramic crowns.

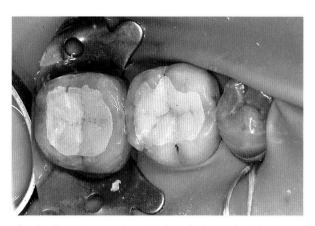

Fig 2–6b Two occlusal inlays being tried in. Note apparent lack of color blend due to air refraction space.

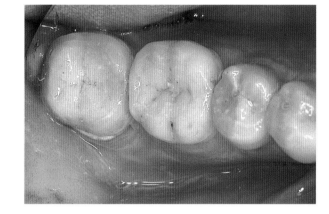

Fig 2–6c Two simple restorations luted in position, restoring stiffness, tooth esthetics, and resistance to abrasion. Note color blend once composite resin is placed under porcelain.

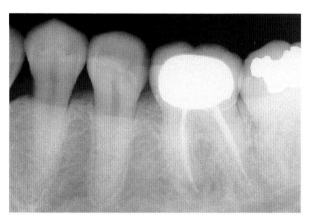

Fig 2–7 Radiograph of compound inlay showing lack of radiopacity.

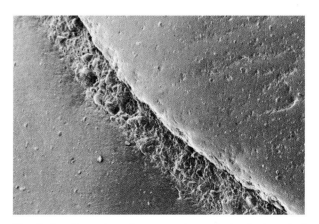

Fig 2–8 Scanning electron micrograph of a bonded restoration luted in position. Note excellence of marginal integrity.

Principles of Porcelain Use as an Inlay/Onlay Material

3

Dan Nathanson

Traditionally, gold has been regarded as the ideal inlay material. As a relatively soft, ductile material, it can be cast with great accuracy and can be further clinically modified by burnishing to be continuous with the margins of the preparation. Gold alloys may exhibit considerable elasti[c] when subjected to a bending test. If the app[lied] stress exceeds the elastic limit, the alloy [may] bend further and exhibit permanent deform[a]tion (bending), but still will not fail (Fig 3–1). These properties make gold an effective material for the fabrication of inlays and onlays.

Porcelain, on the other hand, is a brittle material. One of the main characteristics of a brittle material is the lack of plastic behavior and the inability to withstand plastic deformation under stress. In other words, deformation of (ie, bending) a piece of porcelain beyond its elastic limit (ie, beyond the point at which it acts like a spring) would be "fatal" and the porcelain would break (Figs 3–2 and 3–3). Yet when compressive stress is applied to porcelain that is supported so that bending cannot occur, it can be sustained at high magnitude without failure (Fig 3–4).

Wh[en] dental porcelain is used for the con[struc]tion of a fixed partial denture, normally a [meta]l substructure is used to prevent the porce[lain] from fracturing under the occlusal stress [fr]om the opposing teeth. Without a metal substructure, a porcelain fracture would most probably occur in the pontic area, either at the connectors or through the pontic itself. The metal substructure cannot change the porcelain's mechanical properties and does not give it a different elastic modulus or compressive strength. Instead, if designed properly, the metallic substructure with proper cross-sectional dimensions provides rigidity and resistance to bending that in turn eliminate tensile stresses to the porcelain. This is why only a rigid framework can be successful. A thin, flexible framework can be constructed to sustain the occlusal forces without breaking, but, if any bending occurs, part of the porcelain might be tensed beyond its tensile strength and would ultimately fracture.

Etched porcelain restorations are made of thin ceramic materials and are inherently weaker than metallic restorations. When they are returned to

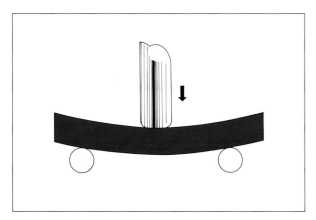

Fig 3–1 Load applied to a metallic test bar in a flexural mode. Bar can sustain initial load in an elastic way. Additional loading beyond the metal's elastic limit will cause bending, but bar will not fail until stress exceeds the ultimate strength of the bar.

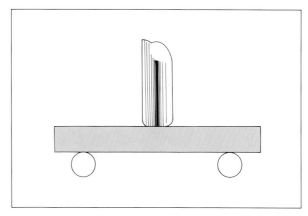

Fig 3–2 Porcelain test bar subjected to a flexural load. To keep porcelain from breaking, load must be limited to within porcelain's elastic limit.

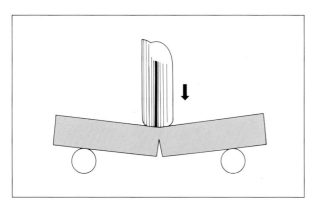

Fig 3–3 When load exceeds the bar's elastic limit, porcelain is unable to bend and fails because it is a brittle material.

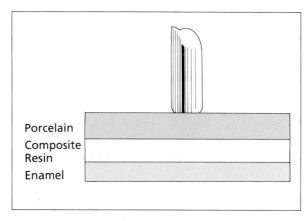

Porcelain
Composite Resin
Enamel

Fig 3–4 Porcelain bar and load identical to those in Fig 3–3. If porcelain is supported with a rigid material, bending is prevented and porcelain does not fail.

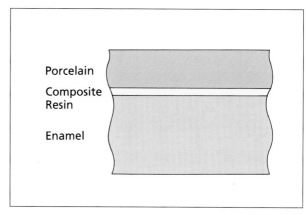

Fig 3–5 Thin porcelain restoration supported by rigid enamel structure via composite resin bonding.

the clinician from the dental laboratory and are tried on the casts and in the oral cavity, a real risk of fracture exists. However, the adhesive bonding of these restorations to teeth produces adequate strength to sustain function and stresses within the oral environment. Without this bonding, even the slight occlusal stresses from the opposing teeth could induce fractures.

The Bonding Mechanism

The improved fracture resistance brought about by the bonding process relies on several mechanisms.

Support by Tooth Structure to Prevent Bending

In a way similar to the way that the metal frame strengthens a porcelain fixed partial denture, the tooth provides the support to keep the porcelain from deforming and fracturing. But just as the porcelain fixed partial denture must be "fused" with the metal framework for the restoration to resist stresses, a posterior porcelain restoration must form a strong bond with the

tooth for the porcelain to be supported. Bonding the porcelain to the tooth's enamel and dentin ensures the stability and integrity that allows tooth structure to provide full support to the otherwise fragile restoration (Fig 3–5). The bonded restoration is protected against displacement and deflection, rendering it resistant to occlusal forces.

Uniform Support and Stress-Relieving Layer

The polymerized composite resin under the bonded porcelain restoration provides a solid support layer of uniform thickness and rigidity. This layer equalizes the variance in elasticity between different tooth structures (ie, between enamel and dentin) and aids by making the underlying support uniform and continuous. It fills minute gaps and provides an adequate zone for relief of potential stresses between the porcelain and underlying tooth structure.

Anti–"Crack Propagation" Forces

Ceramic materials usually fail where small defects are present in the material. These defects, inherent to the porcelain, are caused mainly by internal stressing of the ceramic during processing (ie, contraction during cooling) and are of-

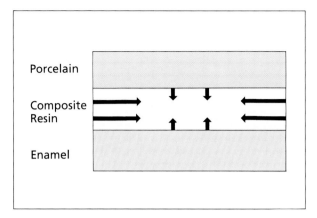

Fig 3–6 Composite resin layer between porcelain restoration and tooth structure is subject to polymerization shrinkage, which is more pronounced in longitudinal direction.

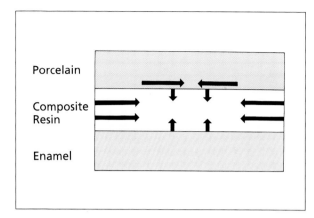

Fig 3–7 Shrinkage of composite resin between porcelain and enamel may counteract crack propagation in porcelain, rendering a ceramic restoration that is resistant to functional stresses in the oral cavity.

ten only microscopic in size. At a molecular level, however, these defects or cracks represent huge gaps, where the molecules on one side of the gap are significantly distant from the molecules on the other side of the gap. This phenomenon can greatly weaken a ceramic material. The greater intermolecular distance across the gap reduces the intermolecular attraction to the extent that relatively low-magnitude tensile stresses would cause the gap to open further and the molecules to be drawn away from each other. This would create a microscopic area of concentrated stress at the bottom of the gap, which in turn would ultimately induce further failure and propagation of the gap.

The described phenomenon can occur in an acute mode, when enough stress is available to induce failure through the material, or in a chronic manner, where fatigue forces (ie, relatively low but repetitive forces) bring about a slowly progressing crack propagation. Either way, the process may lead to a catastrophic failure of the material. The use of a composite resin as a luting agent in conjunction with posterior ceramic restorations introduces an additional porcelain-strengthening mechanism as a result of the composite resin's polymerization shrinkage.

Shrinkage is an inevitable side effect of resin polymerization that is generally viewed as a negative property. However, within certain limits, the composite resin polymerization shrinkage can help strengthen porcelain by exerting a force on the inner porcelain surface that stresses the porcelain molecules together rather than away from each other. This would be in an opposite direction to crack propagation forces (Figs 3–6 and 3–7). The extent of polymerization shrinkage for thin layers of a composite resin agent may in fact be beyond the values reported for the materials in bulk.

Another way to understand the shrinkage effect is to view the porcelain restoration as if it were lined with a uniform layer of composite resin through its inner surface, similar to a porcelain glaze, rendering it more resistant to the rupture effect of tensile forces.

Transfer of Stress to Underlying Structures

A well-bonded ceramic restoration that adheres strongly to the tooth structure forms, in effect, a layer that is an integral part of the tooth, similar to the enamel layer. Enamel in itself is also a brittle structure, but its almost inseparable bond to dentin protects it by transferring external forces all the way into the dentin. This arrangement makes the intact tooth relate to the external forces as one continuous entity, with cross-sectional dimensions and mechanical properties deriving from the combined dentin and enamel layers. Similarly, a well-bonded porcelain inlay or onlay is an integral part of the tooth. Forces applied are transferred through the porcelain to the dentin and theoretically will not cause porcelain failure unless the dentinal layer fails as well. However, if the bonding between the porcelain and tooth is inadequate, the stress will not be transferred further and the porcelain will tend to fracture (similar to unsupported enamel).

Restoration/Preparation Design Requirements

As with other intracoronal restorations, the design parameters of etched ceramic inlays and onlays must take into account the restorative material's properties, strength, and retention requirements. In metallic restorations there is a general positive correlation between the restoration's cross-sectional dimension and its strength. The thicker the metallic restoration, the stronger and the more resistant to deformation and failure it is. This is why silver amalgam restorations with interproximal extensions require adequate depth, especially at the isthmus, and gold onlays should have sufficient gold thickness over the supporting cusp.

The different properties of ceramics dictate different thickness requirements. Ceramic strength is proportional to its cross-sectional thickness only up to a point. Beyond that, added thickness may not add strength and ultimately will reduce strength. Clinicians consider occlusal thicknesses of 1.0 to 2.5 mm to be a safe range for etched porcelain posterior restorations. Uniform thickness may contribute to the success of the restoration.

For a good prognosis, etched porcelain restorations must be well fitted to the prepared teeth. But there is a lesser need to rely on parallel walls and deep boxes than there is for gold inlays. Also, there is no need for a frictional fit as required with metallic inlays or onlays. The avail-ability of a circumferential band of enamel in the prepared tooth would be far more beneficial for retention purposes. Too tight a fit, especially on the buccal and lingual walls, may induce a fracture of the ceramic restoration during the try-in procedure.

Ceramic is brittle, and thin knife-edged margins may easily fracture. The design therefore should include deep chamfer or rounded shoulder margins, to provide a safe thickness and make it easier for the dental technician to handle the restoration. A deep chamfer (as compared to a square shoulder) maintains the benefit of adequate thickness yet enables proper bonding with a larger surface area of etched enamel margins.

Beveling the occlusal cavosurface margin in ceramic inlay preparations is generally not indicated, because the resulting thin ceramic bevel may be vulnerable to occlusal forces.

Temporary Cementing Medium

As with all indirect intracoronal restorations, the posterior ceramic inlay/onlay procedures require adequate provisionalization. Routinely, provisional restorations are made with acrylic resin or autopolymerizing materials. They can be processed intraorally or indirectly on a cast. The well-contoured, anatomically shaped provisional restoration must be cemented with a temporary cement, to allow adequate retention for several weeks and, ultimately, easy removal by the dentist.

For conventional crown-and-bridge procedures, eugenol-containing zinc oxide formulations have been used for years and are still used widely. Resin-cemented etched porcelain restorations, however, require a different kind of temporary cement. The eventual selection of a resin cement for final cementation contraindicates the use of any eugenol-containing temporary cement. Eugenol inhibits the polymerization of resins, and its presence may interfere significantly with the setting of the final cement.

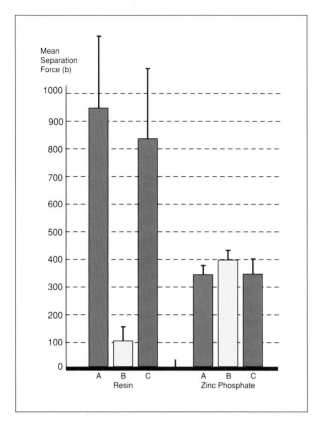

Fig 3–8 Histogram showing separation forces of resin cores cemented with resin and zinc phosphate cements: *(A)* no pretreatment; *(B)* pretreatment with eugenol-containing temporary cement; *(C)* pretreatment with noneugenol temporary cement. (Adapted with permission from Millstein and Nathanson, 1992.)

Table 3–1 *Noneugenol Temporary Cements*

Material	Manufacturer	Address
Temp-Bond NE	Kerr Mfg	28200 Wick Rd., Box 455, Romulus, MI 48174 (800) 537-7123
Nogenol	GC America	3737 West 127th St. Chicago, IL 60658 (800) 323-7063
Zone	Cadco Dental Products	600 East Hueneme Rd. Oxnard, CA 93033 (800) 833-8267
Proviscell	Septodont, Inc	PO Box 11926 Wilmington, DE 19850 (800) 872-8305

A study of the retention of metal rings to metallic cores using a urethane resin cement and zinc oxiphosphate cement (Millstein and Nathanson, 1983) showed that significantly better retention was achieved with resin cement. However, the results were different when the metal cores were first cemented to the rings with a eugenol temporary cement, then separated, cleaned, and recemented with either urethane resin or zinc oxiphosphate. The eugenol traces caused a dramatic reduction in retention with the urethane resin cement but had no effect on the zinc oxiphosphate (Fig 3–8).

This experiment with metal fixtures clearly identifies the contraindication of using eugenol cements prior to cementation with a resin. Intraorally, the effect may be even more pronounced, since tooth structure, with its rougher and more porous surface, can retain the eugenol better than can the experimental metal cores. Although this phenomenon has not been fully confirmed in clinical situations, it would be prudent in such applications to limit the use of temporary cement to products that do not include eugenol in their formulation. A partial list of such products is provided in Table 3–1. Even with these materials, correct protocol should call for thorough cleaning of the preparation walls (ie, with fine pumice) prior to final cementation to remove all traces of temporary cement that may have adhered to the tooth.

Tooth Preparation

4

The advent of etched enamel, resin-bonded restorations has changed the general concepts of tooth preparation advocated years ago by G. V. Black. The newer preparation designs need no longer adhere to the principles of "extension for prevention," so that the marginal areas are not necessarily brought out into "self-cleansing" regions of the tooth. In this type of restoration, tooth reduction becomes considerably more conservative, because the bonding procedures and resultant sealing to enamel provide ongoing **prevention, without the need for extension**, as well as retention in even the shallowest of preparations. The premise of tooth preparation for etched porcelain inlays/onlays is therefore a modification of these original tenets, retaining the principles of resistance form but eliminating the need for developing a specific retention form or "extension for prevention."

The typical amalgam restoration requires a certain dimension of tooth reduction irrespective of the extent of preexisting tooth destruction. This is to accommodate the inherent weakness of the amalgam or even gold in thin sections. **Etched porcelain can be bonded to existing tooth structure in sections thinner than 2 mm**, thereby negating this need for additional tooth reduction to satisfy the inadequacies of other restorative materials.

The amalgam or cast-gold preparation must often be similarly extended into healthy tooth structure to develop retention form for the restoration. The walls of these preparations are made slightly "off-parallel" for frictional retention. In today's era of the bonded restoration, the adhesive nature of the "etched porcelain/composite resin/tooth complex" radically alters this approach.

It is simply no longer necessary to develop frictional retention; in fact, it is contraindicated.

In the classic amalgam or cast-gold restoration, it is also necessary to remove any undermined enamel because this unsupported tooth structure tends to fracture. The bonded restoration offers various alternatives in that, even if the undercut is within the confines of dentin, this undercut area can be blocked out with a glass-ionomer cement buildup prior to final preparation and impressions. Alternatively, it can be blocked out in the laboratory on the die prior to the fabrication of the etched porcelain restoration. During the seating procedure this space will be filled and bonded with the composite resin luting agent, restoring cuspal stiffness and strength to the entire tooth. This strengthening effect is caused by the dual bonding of the composite resin to the tooth enamel and to the etched silanated porcelain restorations, thus not only providing support for the compromised cusp but also effectively sealing the margins.

Modifications in Preparation Design

The properties and laboratory requirements for fabrication of porcelain restorations require certain modifications to the preparations used for cast restorations. First, G. V. Black's original concepts for restorations demanded sharp, definitive line angles, which are obviously contraindicated in any form of porcelain restoration. Therefore, *all line and point angles are of necessity rounded* (Fig 4–1). This is to facilitate the laboratory fabrication of the porcelain restoration and to decrease the potential for these areas to propagate as fractures within the restorative complex.

Second, unlike cast-metal inlays and onlays, the etched porcelain inlay requires *no classic bevel* to aid in the sealing of these restorations. In the etched porcelain restoration, the void between the tooth and the inlay is filled with a relatively insoluble composite resin luting agent that bonds to both the tooth and the porcelain, thus sealing the complex more effectively than the traditional cement line. The classic bevel is, in fact, contraindicated because it will necessitate the fabrication of a thin edge of porcelain so friable it will tend to fracture during trial placement of the restorations. There is evidence, however, that a *hollow-ground chamfer* confined to the marginal enamel will aid in developing a more effective seal (Fig 4–2). This is due to exposure of enamel rods at right angles to the finish line. This porcelain extension will also help develop a blend in color as it overlies the tooth substance below, making the demarcation line between tooth or porcelain imperceptible. This is facilitated in the laboratory by adding increments of translucent porcelain to this area, permitting more of the underlying tooth color to bleed through the porcelain and reach the surface.

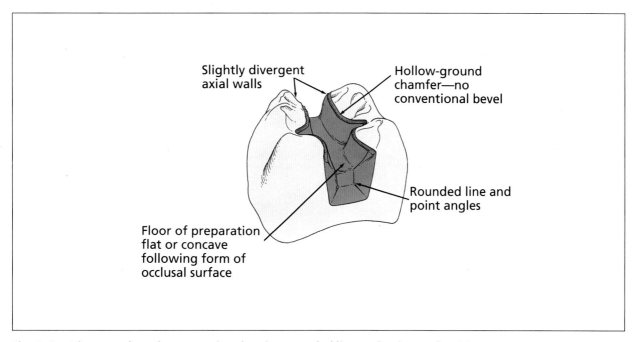

Slightly divergent axial walls

Hollow-ground chamfer—no conventional bevel

Rounded line and point angles

Floor of preparation flat or concave following form of occlusal surface

Fig 4–1 Diagram of tooth preparation showing rounded line and point angles, 15-degree divergent walls, and hollow-ground chamfer at periphery of occlusal surface.

The basic premise of the etched porcelain preparation is conservatism: preservation of all that remains; restoration of form, function, and strength to the tooth; and long-term maintenance of these features.

Only those aspects of the tooth already compromised by caries or trauma are reshaped to facilitate the fabrication of a porcelain restoration to replace these missing aspects. Slight modifications are permitted to develop better resistance form, plus a peripheral hollow-ground chamfer. This should restore not only form and function but also esthetics to the tooth, protect the tooth, and eliminate further breakdown.

Clinical Principles of Tooth Preparation

Removal of Old Restorations and/or Caries

It is preferable to remove any existing restorations and compromised tooth structure before deciding on the definitive form of the preparation and final restoration. Old restorations may be removed more easily before placement of the rubber dam. The open contacts in compound cavity preparations facilitate quicker placement of the rubber dam. Existing liners or bases should also be judiciously removed at this stage, leaving merely sound tooth structure in place. If there are no previous restorations, only caries is removed.

Isolation

The teeth involved should be isolated with a rubber dam before a specific form is developed for the preparation. This makes it easier to visualize the ultimate configuration of the restoration and provides moisture control during placement of any required bases. With the rubber dam in place, any remaining infected or softened dentin should be removed, and the affected dentin should be checked to see whether it will compromise the new restoration in any way. When esthetics is a major consideration,

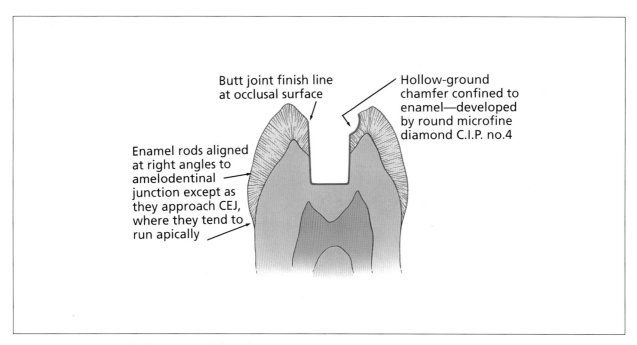

Butt joint finish line at occlusal surface

Hollow-ground chamfer confined to enamel—developed by round microfine diamond C.I.P. no.4

Enamel rods aligned at right angles to amelodentinal junction except as they approach CEJ, where they tend to run apically

Fig 4–2 Diagram of hollow-ground chamfer used to expose an increased number of enamel rods for increased bond strength, increased marginal seal, and a transition for better esthetic color blend.

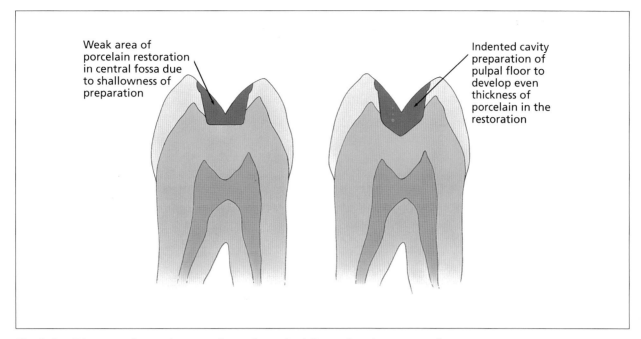

Weak area of porcelain restoration in central fossa due to shallowness of preparation

Indented cavity preparation of pulpal floor to develop even thickness of porcelain in the restoration

Fig 4–3   Diagram of two alternate forms for pulpal floor of cavity preparation; form is dependent on cavity depth.

dentin discolored by caries or by amalgam may need to be removed, even if it is otherwise sound. Dentin that is stained, but not infected, on the pulpal floor is generally not of any great consequence, as it can easily be opaqued.

The cavity form, by its very nature, is developed as conservatively as possible; only the compromised portion of the tooth is removed and convenient access is provided for the subsequent porcelain restoration.

Components of Preparation Design

Pulpal Floor. The pulpal floor should be developed, by a combination of calculated, judicious tooth reduction and a fortified glass-ionomer cement base, into a surface with definitive resistance form. This is probably relevant to the long-term success of the restoration because it decreases the shearing forces on the composite resin–luting agent interface. The cohesive bonds in the luting agent can hydrolyze and weaken over time because of stress and thermal cycling. The cavity design should also facilitate laboratory fabrication and ensure specific localization of the restoration during placement.

The configuration of this pulpal floor can vary according to the depth of the preparation (Fig 4–3). It need not be classically flat and perpendicular to the long axis of the tooth, as required for cast-gold restorations. If the cavity is shallow, this will result in a weak area in the central fossa of the restoration. In such situations, *the pulpal floor should be indented in the central fossa region to parallel the cuspal inclines,* resulting in a thickness of porcelain in the center that is similar to that on the lateral aspects of the restoration.

Axial Walls. The axial walls of the cavity preparation should be slightly more divergent from the pulpal floor toward the enamel surface than would be prepared for a conventional cast-metal inlay, where the 6- to 10-degree taper is commonly favored to develop retention. The use of adhesive composite resin luting agents negates the need for parallelism and frictional fit for retention. The *increased taper* of the axial walls allows easier placement and removal of the restoration during the try-in phase, but the taper should not be exaggerated so as to unnecessarily remove additional tooth structure.

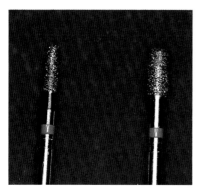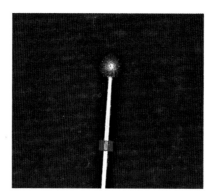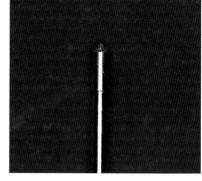

Fig 4–4   C.I.P. two-grit diamond (Brasseler Corp) with fine grit on the tip and a rounded radius and medium-grit hybrid up the shank.

Figs 4–5a and b   *(a)* Round microfine diamond for developing the hollow-ground chamfer. *(b)* The C.I.P. no. 4 diamond for developing the indented central fossa.

Finish Line. The occlusal cavosurface margin of the restoration *should not be beveled*, because it is difficult to fire porcelain to such a thin section, which would also have the potential to fracture during seating. There are two schools of thought on the actual configuration of the finish line. It may be developed as *(1)* **a well-defined, smooth butt joint** or *(2)* **a hollow-ground chamfer** (see Fig 4–2).

The hollow-ground chamfer appears to be preferable (see Fig 4–2), because it creates a more effective seal for the restoration and improves esthetic color blending. These properties are due to the configuration of the margin and the pattern of the enamel prisms made available for etching over an extended enamel border. It also aids in esthetically blending the junction of tooth and restoration by allowing the underlying tooth color to bleed through this semitranslucent section of porcelain, making this interface imperceptible.

In a proximal box, because of the proximity of the cementoenamel junction to the finish line, it is desirable to have a flat floor ending on enamel to maximize sealing potential.

Internal Line Angles. The typically well-defined internal line and point angles of cast-metal restorations are of necessity rounded for porcelain. The preparation is therefore performed with a specifically designed tapered cylinder that has a flat end with a rounded radius (Fig 4–4). The concept of a dual-grit diamond (Two-Grit Ceramic Inlay Preparation System [C.I.P.], Brasseler Corp) has been found to be most effective in ceramic restorations. This unique instrument has a fine-grit diamond on the tip for 0.5 mm up the shank and a coarser-grit diamond up the rest of the shank. The instrument therefore tends to cut less aggressively pulpally, reducing the potential for overpreparation, particularly on a glass-ionomer base, which reduces more easily than tooth substance.

The specifically developed instrument with a newly designed tip results in the following:

- A flat pulpal floor with the calculated divergent axial walls
- A rounded line angle between the pulpal and axial wall
- Highly retentive axial walls because of the hybrid diamond on the shank, which increases the surface area for bonding and develops mechanical retention
- A well-defined cavosurface margin at the occlusal surface on which the hollow-ground chamfer can be developed (best accomplished with a fine-grit round instrument [eg, C.I.P. no. 5 or 6, Brasseler Corp]) (Fig 4–5)

Specific Modifications for Different Types of Cavity Preparations

Class II Restorations

When the carious lesion on a tooth encompasses the approximal portion as well as the occlusal surface, a compound two- to three-surface restoration becomes necessary. If the lesion only involves the approximal surface below the contact point, an alternative such as the "tunnel" procedure with glass-ionomer cement and composite resin may be possible (Fig 4–6). Contact relations, cuspal stiffness, and hence tooth strength are best maintained by not incorporating the marginal ridge unless necessary.

The Class II restoration can best be described for a tooth with occlusal and approximal caries or with previous compound restorations (Fig 4–7). Old restorations should be removed before a rubber dam is placed for isolation and to improve access and visualization (Fig 4–8). The outline should encompass only those grooves and fossae that show evidence of caries.

The occlusal surface is then extended by using the same C.I.P. no. 1 instrument until the bur reaches the marginal ridge. It is moved at right angles to the central fossa just within the proximal marginal ridge. The proximal box is progressively developed to the depth of the base of the caries gingivally and extended until contact is almost broken laterally (buccally and lingually) or to the lateral extent of the decay. A sharp enamel chisel can be used to break through this contact area to avoid damaging the adjacent tooth. The judicious use of a finely tapered microfine diamond or carbide finishing instrument (eg, E.T., Brasseler Corp) will do the same. The adjacent teeth can also be wedged apart to allow for easier access when the approximal region is prepared.

If the contact area is wide in a buccolingual dimension, as occurs between two molars, it may not be necessary to extend the cavity preparation buccally and lingually; it may be possible to limit it to the lateral extent of the caries within the confines of the contact area. This is most relevant when caries is nominal and the development of a classic box form will remove additional unaffected tooth structure.

If there is a preexisting failing restoration, this should be removed entirely (Fig 4–8). The remaining tooth is examined with a view *to developing definitive resistance form, a path of insertion, and finish lines* using the C.I.P. no. 2 (see Fig 4–11). The walls of the box should diverge slightly to facilitate easy placement of the restoration without binding. The line angle where the occlusal aspect of the preparation joins the proximal-axial wall should be well rounded and the two surfaces blended into one another.

The curvature of the facial and lingual walls of the box are modified to be flat, thus eliminating undercuts, and to facilitate placement of the restoration. If the other approximal surfaces are similarly involved, the approach to the preparation of the box will be similar.

The pulpal floor can be a shallow V-shape down the central fossa line to develop a more even thickness of porcelain in the final restoration. The two-grit I.P.S. no. 4 (see Fig 4–5) will do this automatically. The floor should have an even depth of 1.5 to 2.5 mm, except in areas where there is evidence of deeper caries. These areas can be filled in to level the floor using a light-cured base (Figs 4–9 and 4–10).

A hollow-ground chamfer is created at the occlusal finish line using a fine-grit round diamond C.I.P. no. 3 (Fig 4–12). The completed preparation (Fig 4–13) is ready for impression making.

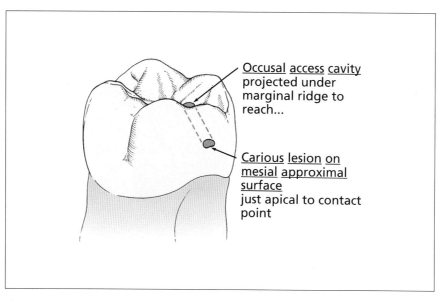

Occusal access cavity
projected under
marginal ridge to
reach...

Carious lesion on
mesial approximal
surface
just apical to contact
point

Fig 4–6 Diagram of the tunnel procedure for small approximal carious lesions without any occlusal surface involvement. Glass-ionomer restorative medium is used to fill the tunnel. This is subsequently removed from the occlusal aspect, where appropriately colored composite resin is placed. Note retention of marginal ridge, contact relations, and original approximal contours.

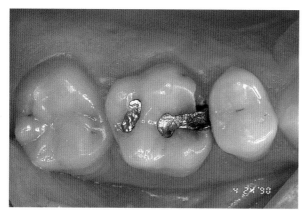

Fig 4–7 Preoperative occlusal view of a maxillary first molar with two failing amalgam restorations.

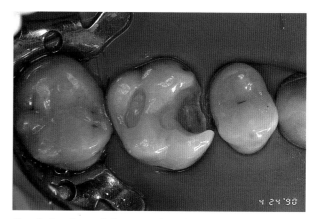

Fig 4–8 Remaining tooth substance following removal of old restoration and preexisting recurrent caries. The tooth is isolated with a rubber dam prior to any refining of the cavity preparation.

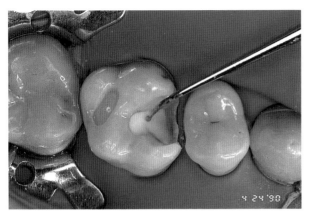

Fig 4–9 Vitrebond glass-ionomer cement base (3M Dental) is placed with the NovaTech PiNT 11 to develop resistance form, line out undercuts, even the depth of the pulpal floor, and cover all exposed dentin

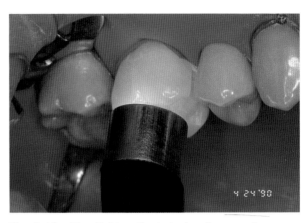

Fig 4–10 The light-activated glass-ionomer/composite resin base is cured.

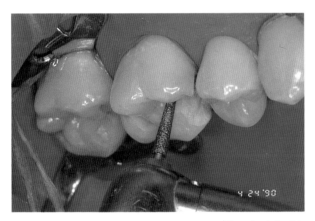

Fig 4–11 The cavity preparation is refined with the C.I.P. no. 2 bur.

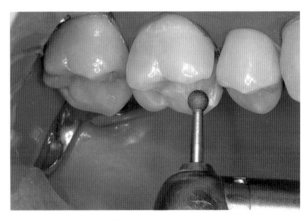

Fig 4–12 The hollow-ground chamfer is developed as the occlusal finish line using the C.I.P. no. 3.

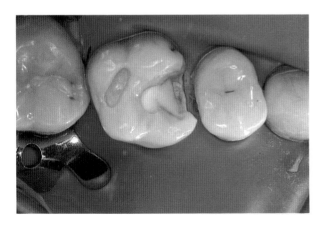

Fig 4–13 Completed cavity preparation ready for impression making.

Inlays Versus Onlays

The etched porcelain posterior restoration is a relatively new concept, and, as such, there are few specific guidelines as to when an inlay should become an onlay. The adhesive nature of the bonded restoration makes unnecessary the traditional approach of additional preparation to protect unsupported cusps or to develop resistance and retention form (Fig 4–14a). *In fact, removal of additional tooth structure to onlay cusps is contraindicated, because it will often result in a porcelain cusp in occlusal contact with the opposing central fossa.* Maintaining the restoration intracoronally may well retain the centric hold with the opposing arch in natural tooth substance and decrease the potential for wear — without decreasing the overall strength.

If an onlay is necessary, the occlusal scheme should be developed so that during lateral excursions of the mandible minimal or no contact is made with the porcelain. The restoration functions occlusally predominantly as a centric hold. Obviously this is not always possible, but it is certainly desirable and is achieved by decreasing the functional outer aspect of the ceramic supporting cusp. As such it may be difficult to ensure that this ceramic functional outer aspect does not traverse the natural tooth substance of the opposing dentition in lateral excursive movements of the mandible, creating wear facets.

In general then, the preparation should remain as conservative as possible, but at the same time *it is desirable not to have the porcelain restoration–tooth interface in an area where it is constantly subjected to heavy occlusal forces.*

These forces result in wear of the composite resin luting agent and potential fracture of the enamel at the cavosurface margin. This "ditching" effect must be minimized or an onlay may be preferable.

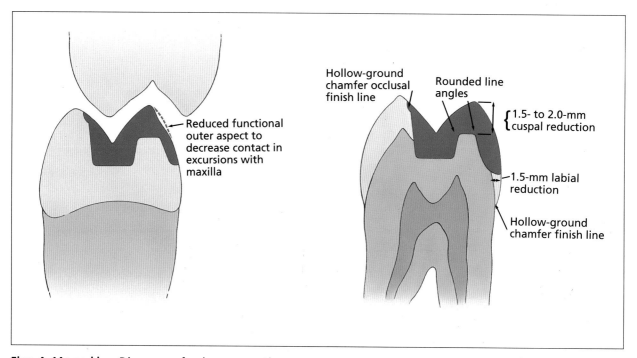

Figs 4–14a and b   Diagrams of onlay preparation.

Cuspal Onlay Preparation

In those situations where a cusp is fractured or previously restored, it becomes necessary to incorporate it into the final form of the restoration.

The preparation should incorporate the following features (Fig 4–14b):

- A 1.5- to 2.0-mm reduction in vertical height of the cusps and all occluding areas
- Preparation finish lines on any supporting cusps that are hollow-ground chamfers, generally with *no bevel*
- Well-rounded angles on the cuspal preparation, to prevent propagation of porcelain fracture from these sharp stress points

The premise of the preparation is to allow the fabrication of a porcelain restoration that has *as simple a geometric form as possible,* yet has the wherewithal to support the tooth with *definitive resistance form* (Figs 4–15 to 4–22).

Slot Preparation for Approximal Caries

If approximal caries extends well into the dentin, undermining the marginal ridge areas to the extent that a tunnel preparation with glass-ionomer cement and composite resin becomes nonviable, then the slot preparation may be an alternative. This preparation incorporates the marginal ridge and proximal surface but not the complete occlusal surface; thus it is an esthetic, conservative alternative to full-coverage or compound cast-metal restorations.

The C.I.P. no. 1 diamond is then used to judiciously remove the undermined marginal ridge area and extend this box form laterally to the extent of the lesion buccally, lingually, and pulpally. The box form should be mildly divergent, gingivoocclusally, and can be either in the form of a dovetail or a flared box, depending on the extent of the caries and outline form of the tooth. It is not necessary for the cavity preparation to extend into the so-called self-cleansing areas, either buccally or lingually, and the preparation can, in fact, remain within the confines of the contact area if necessary. Placement procedures should then involve the use of the separating wedge to facilitate access to the porcelain-tooth interface, so that the excess composite resin flash can be removed and the interface polished to a high, non-plaque-retentive luster.

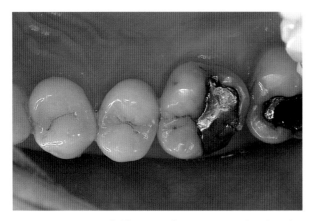

Fig 4–15 Large failing amalgam restoration involving distal two thirds of maxillary molar.

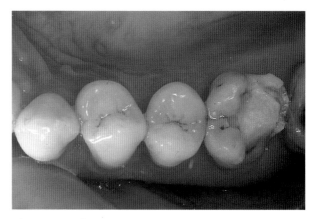

Fig 4–16 The restoration is removed, as is recurrent caries, and the dentin is covered with a glass-ionomer base before final preparation. Note that the mesial aspect of the tooth is not given an onlay preparation (ie, all uncompromised tooth structure is retained).

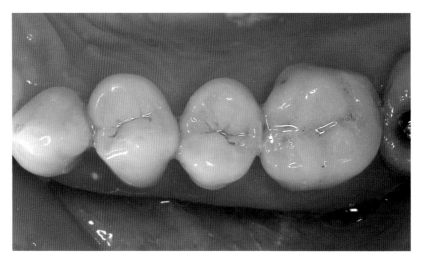

Fig 4–17 Postoperative view of inlay/onlay luted in position.

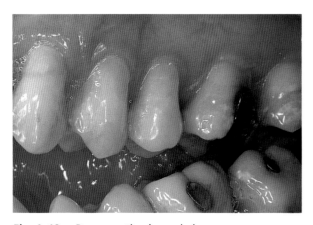

Fig 4–18 Preoperative buccal view.

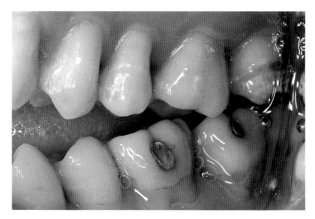

Fig 4–19 Postoperative buccal view.

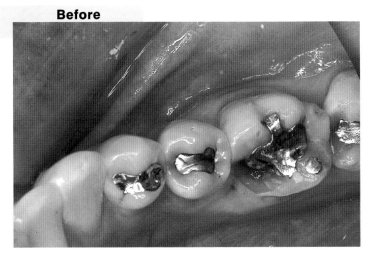

Fig 4–20 Failing amalgam restoration.

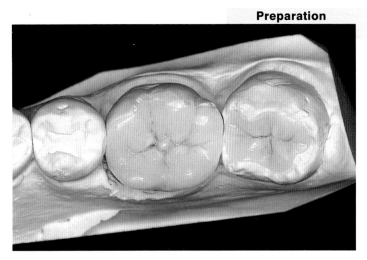

Fig 4–21 Ceramic restorations on model.

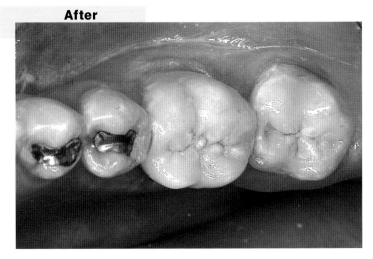

Fig 4–22 Postoperative view of onlay in position.

Class III Inlays

There are few indications for this type of etched porcelain inlay. However, it is useful in moderate to extensive Class III restorations on anterior teeth where the approach has been via the lingual surface, thus leaving the buccal surface esthetically uncompromised. An etched porcelain inlay will provide support for the remaining tooth structure when deemed necessary, particularly where contact relations are difficult to develop because of the large size of the preparation. Etched porcelain inlays thus provide a viable and conservative alternative to the full-coverage restoration.

Following are additional indications for the Class III etched porcelain inlay:

- Large amalgam or composite resin restorations involving the mesial or distolingual surface of a canine may show unacceptable discoloration or compromised contact relations (Fig 4–23).
- In lateral excursive movements of the mandible, the mandibular teeth may traverse the lingual aspect of a large composite resin restoration or existing caries, and there may be a need to restore effective anterior guidance using a bonded porcelain restoration. (If the opposing contact relation is on a natural tooth, wear against the porcelain restoration is a potential problem.)
- A heavily undermined incisal edge or approximal surface on an incisor may require support to prevent an otherwise esthetic tooth from fracturing.

Preparation Form. The Class III preparation is similar to the basic slot preparation for any cast-metal restoration. The proximal box is started from the lingual surface with a pear-shaped carbide bur to penetrate to the depth of the decay. The C.I.P. no. 2 diamond is inserted into this access cavity and extended incisally or gingivally within the confines of the contact area to develop an outline form limited to the lateral extent of the caries or old restoration (Fig 4–24).

Any remaining unsupported enamel at the contact area is removed with a chisel or E.T. carbide, and the enamel curvature on the gingival and incisal walls of the box are flattened with the same chisel to provide a path of insertion without undercuts. This can effectively be done with a tapered finishing carbide (eg, E.T. no. 6, Brasseler Corp).

It is important not to extend the preparation any further incisally, gingivally, or pulpally than is absolutely essential to remove the caries and provide access. The outline form is merely a convenience form and is predicated on: (1) the extent of the lesion, (2) the need to develop a path of insertion, and (3) the technical demands of the ceramist to facilitate easier laboratory fabrication.

The walls of the box should diverge to facilitate a path of insertion for the restoration from the lingual aspect toward the buccal aspect (Fig 4–25).

Example of Class III Inlay

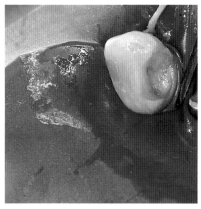

Fig 4–23 Preparation outline form. Note there is no bevel or hollow-ground chamfer, because of lack of space and because there is no need for esthetic blend in a lingual aspect.

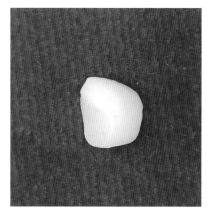

Fig 4–24 Class III ceramic distal lingual inlay.

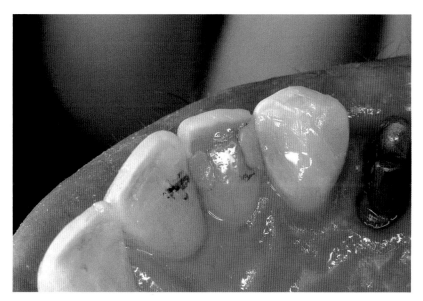

Fig 4–25 Postoperative lingual view of inlay luted in position.

Class IV Inlays

Class IV inlays have been shown to be a most effective use of the porcelain inlay. The porcelain will replace the missing incisal and/or proximal aspects of the tooth and is considerably stronger than a similar restoration fabricated in composite resin. The preparation involves removal of any remaining decay and smoothing of the fracture line at right angles to the buccal and lingual surfaces of the tooth (Figs 4–26 and 4–27). The enamel finish line of the buccal surface of the tooth is then developed into a bevel or, if the enamel is thick enough, a hollow-ground chamfer. The lingual surface is prepared as a butt joint (or a mini-chamfer in the case of a maxillary tooth).

If the buccal finish line is along the bevel, it will be extremely difficult to fire porcelain to this configuration. Hence, the porcelain is baked into a thicker section (Figs 4–28 and 4–29) and then ground back level with the tooth surface, resulting in an imperceptible junction of tooth and porcelain (Fig 4–30).

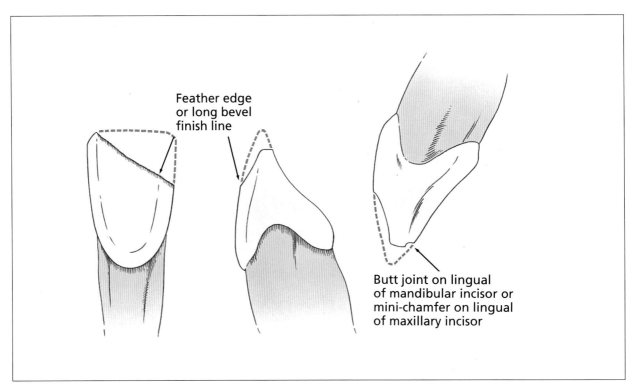

Feather edge or long bevel finish line

Butt joint on lingual of mandibular incisor or mini-chamfer on lingual of maxillary incisor

Fig 4–26 Diagram of Class IV preparation form.

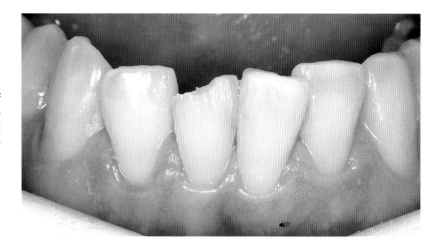

Fig 4–27 Preoperative views of Class IV fracture. Preparation consists of a long bevel on the buccal aspect and butt joint on the lingual aspect of the tooth.

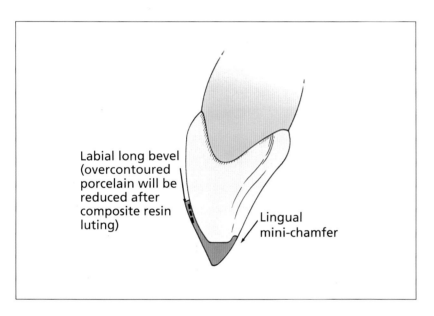

Labial long bevel (overcontoured porcelain will be reduced after composite resin luting)

Lingual mini-chamfer

Fig 4–28 Diagram of the way in which porcelain is formed into a thicker section on the labial bevel and, following placement, is ground level with the tooth surface.

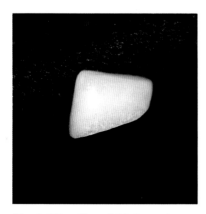

Fig 4–29 Class IV inlay prior to luting.

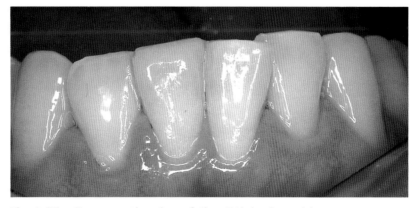

Fig 4–30 Postoperative view of Class IV inlay in position.

Cavity Bases

Glass-Ionomer Materials

Glass-ionomer materials are manufactured in three distinct forms, each of which has very different properties:

1. Type I: luting agents. Type I glass-ionomer cements have a high degree of flow, low viscosity, and thin film thickness, making them useful as cementing media. They have an extended working time and an easier set than do Types II and III. Although they are excellent for use as cements, they are considerably weaker than other types and therefore are not useful as bases or as buildups under porcelain restorations.
2. Type II: restorative materials. Type II glass-ionomer materials are the strongest of the three types, and as such they have a somewhat delayed setting time. They can be mixed with various other metals to develop *cermet* restorative materials. The addition of precious metals has been proposed as a means of adding to the strength of the material (Wilson and McLean, 1988).
3. Type III: bases and liners. Type III glass-ionomer materials are designed to set more rapidly to facilitate their use as bases and liners. This tends to result in a relative decrease in strength, but the strength is usually adequate for non-stress-bearing restorations.

    The addition of composite resin enhances the strength and properties of this material.

Clinical Parameters for Use of Glass-Ionomer Bases

Conventional glass-ionomer materials should be used in thicknesses greater than 1.5 mm in any situation where they will be subsequently etched. A thinner layer will dissolve during etching, resulting in crazing and microcracks. If this occurs, the glass-ionomer base will no longer serve as a protective barrier for the dentin. When a large amount of dentin is to be replaced with a glass-ionomer base, a Type II restorative material or metal-reinforced (ie, cermet cement) or composite resin–reinforced glass-ionomer material should be used.

If the cavity preparation is shallow and has only one or two localized areas of dentinal excavation, one of the more rapidly setting Type III glass-ionomer bases can be used. These bases may also be used to fill out localized depressions in the dentin when the cavity is shallow enough to preclude the use of a glass-ionomer base over the rest of the pulpal floor. In these situations, the restoration should be luted with one of the third-generation dentin bonding agents to seal and bond the composite resin cementing medium to the unlined portions of dentin.

The opacity of glass-ionomer bases can affect the final color of the restoration; therefore, an appropriate shade that will blend in with the adjacent teeth should be selected.

Glass-ionomer based materials have been suggested as the material of choice to replace missing dentin in large preparations or to redevelop a more desirable resistance form in those situations where localized caries has made the preparation floor uneven. The glass-ionomer materials were advocated for the following reasons:

- The glass-ionomer adheres to the dentin via a process of molecular bonding, and this base, when set, can in turn be etched to provide for mechanical retention via a composite resin luting agent.
- Glass-ionomer materials appear to have a high degree of biocompatibility and apparently cause only a transitory inflammatory pulpal tissue response. Resolution of this inflammatory response appears to take place within the first 35 days, and the set cement causes no increase in secondary dentin formation. This is an important factor, because the glass-ionomer cement must be in intimate contact with the dentin for the process of molecular adhesive bonding to take place.
- Glass-ionomer bases have ongoing anticariogenic properties because of the leaching of fluoride.
- The material has good adhesive properties and dimensional stability, so that an accurately fitted restoration can be seated.
- Glass-ionomer bases have reasonably high compressive strengths (up to 200 MPa) but somewhat weak flexural strengths (5 to 40 MPa). Hence, they are relatively effective in confined areas such as bases but are poor as extensive restorations (Wilson and McLean, 1988).

The addition of a composite resin to glass-ionomer has made the base material considerably stronger and more resistant to flexural forces. The combination material is then light cured, which gives it immediate strength.

The physical properties of conventional glass-ionomer bases make them technique-sensitive. They are hydrophilic and susceptible to fluid exposure until the final set has taken place. The adhesive bond to tooth is a molecular or chemical bond, unlike the mechanical bond seen in etched enamel–composite resin bonding. Fortunately, some of this bond strength is attained within the first 30 minutes after placement, but the full adhesion develops over several days.

In the light-cured combination glass-ionomer–composite resin bases, the initial "set" involves bonding of the composite resin as it is exposed to light. This reinforces the glass-ionomer cement and protects it during this early phase of curing. Subsequent bonding of the composite resin lut-ing agent to a glass-ionomer base is achieved by etching the glass-ionomer base with orthophosphoric acid (37%) for less than 8 seconds. This process partially dissolves the matrix, creating a roughened surface with irregularities and crevices into which the composite resin is allowed to penetrate, forming the usual retentive mechanical tags. Studies have shown that the bond strength of composite resin to glass-ionomer bases exceeds the cohesive strength of the conventional glass-ionomer itself (Wilson and McLean, 1988).

If the cavity is not that extensive, it is preferable not to use a glass-ionomer base but to bond directly to the dentin with one of the newer dentin bonding agents.

Small indentations in the pulpal floor can be filled in with a light-cured glass-ionomer base, leaving the rest of the dentin exposed and available for direct bonding.

Impressions and Provisional Restorations

5

Porcelain laminate veneers require no period of provisionalization, but the provisionalization stage is essential with etched porcelain inlays/onlays. This is to ensure that, following preparation and impression making, no change takes place in the position of the prepared or adjacent tooth (ie, no mesial or distal movement of the prepared teeth or supereruption of its antagonist).

The provisional restoration should both stabilize the existing occlusal relationships and protect the prepared teeth from any noxious stimuli.

Depending on the number of teeth involved, the provisional restorations can be made before or after impression making. In general, when multiple units are to be restored, *it is better to fabricate the provisional restorations prior to impression making.* This allows the clinician the opportunity to ascertain whether reduction of all aspects of the preparation is adequate and even, thus providing for subsequent even thicknesses of the porcelain restoration. Provisionalization prior to impression making also allows the direct fabrication of the restoration in the mouth, where the inadvertent contact of a preparation margin with a finishing bur will then not compromise the final restoration.

The type of provisional restoration that should be used will depend on the number of teeth being prepared and the size of the preparation. There are three basic systems for fabricating provisional restorations: *(1)* direct method, *(2)* indirect method, and *(3)* combination direct-indirect method. Either self-curing acrylic resin or light-activated composite resin can be used; each has its relative merits, indications, and contraindications.

Direct-Indirect Method

Self-Curing Acrylic Resin Provisional Restoration With a Vacuform Shell or Preoperative Alginate Impression

This is a standard technique used for conventional crown-and-bridge prosthodontics, in which self-curing acrylic resin is mixed into a somewhat soupy state and flowed into the prepared teeth

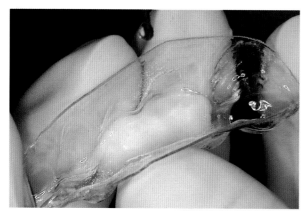

Fig 5–1 The acrylic resin is placed in a clear vacuform matrix before it is placed over the prepared teeth.

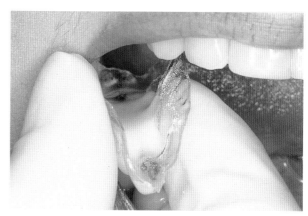

Fig 5–2 The vacuform matrix is manipulated into position over the prepared teeth and allowed to cure only partially.

in a vacuform matrix or preoperative alginate impression (Fig 5–1). This acrylic resin is allowed to cure until the surface sheen is lost and the resin reaches a doughy stage. At this point, the vacuform matrix or impression is manipulated into position over the prepared teeth (Fig 5–2), which have been lubricated to facilitate removal of the impression.

After an initial period of setting, but before the acrylic resin hardens, the vacuform matrix containing the provisional restorations is manipulated on and off the prepared teeth while the acrylic resin undergoes its final curing phase. This procedure keeps the acrylic resin from engaging in any undercuts and allows easy removal once the provisional restoration has cured completely. It also decreases the potential for pulpal irritation caused by the heat generated during the curing process. It is useful to combine this procedure with an intermittent water spray from the chip syringe.

Once the acrylic resin is set, the vacuform matrix is removed from the mouth with the acrylic resin provisional restoration within. The excess acrylic resin is trimmed back to the margins with a laboratory acrylic resin bur (Figs 5–3 and 5–4).

It is more convenient, when a series of adjacent teeth is being restored, not to make individual units but to leave the inlays in one contiguous piece. This facilitates manipulation, trimming, and cementation of the provisional restoration. It also ensures maintenance of the interproximal contact relations and stability of the tooth-to-tooth relations.

The contiguous series of trimmed provisional inlays is returned to the mouth, tried in, and checked for fit and marginal integrity. Any occlusal adjustments in both centric and lateral excursive movements of the mandible are now performed. If any of the margins are grossly inaccurate, it may be necessary to institute a relining procedure. (However, because of the small amount of acrylic resin within an inlay preparation, compared to the amount in a complete-crown restoration, the marginal distortion is considerably smaller and usually within clinically acceptable limits.) If, however, a margin must be added over a reduced cusp in an onlay preparation, it is easiest to accomplish by adding acrylic resin powder and liquid, with a small, sable-hair paintbrush, to a monomer-moistened acrylic resin margin.

The adjusted provisional restorations are removed from the mouth, so that they can be further trimmed and the occlusal anatomy can be developed within the nominal confines of the resin. If desired, they can then be characterized and stained with acrylic stain (eg, with Lang Jet Adjusters or Taub Minute stains) to blend in with the adjacent teeth (Fig 5–5). The provisional restoration is placed (Fig 5–6) with a non–eu-

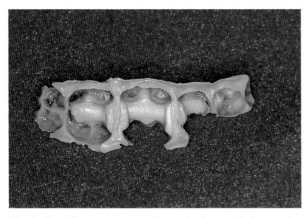

Fig 5–3 The excess acrylic resin beyond the cavity margin is trimmed back to the finish line with an acrylic resin bur.

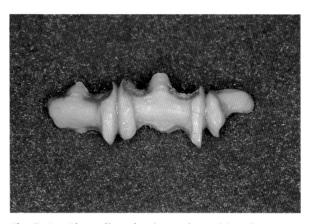

Fig 5–4 The splinted, trimmed provisional restorations are opened interproximally to accommodate interdental soft tissues.

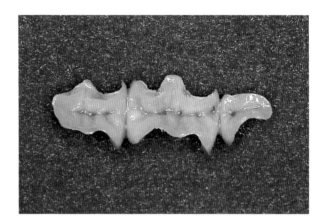

Fig 5–5 The provisional restoration is finally contoured and, if desired, can be characterized and stained.

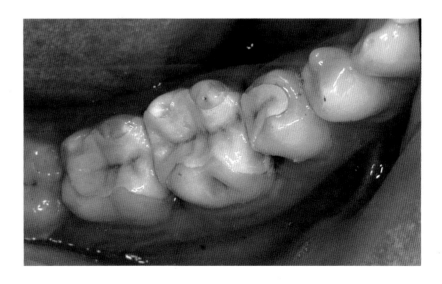

Fig 5–6 The provisional restoration is tried in and checked for marginal fit, interproximal contact, and occlusal relationships. Buccal cavity to be filled with composite resin.

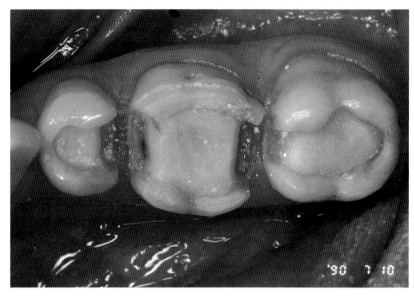

Fig 5–7 Two inlay preparations and an onlay preparation for etched porcelain restorations.

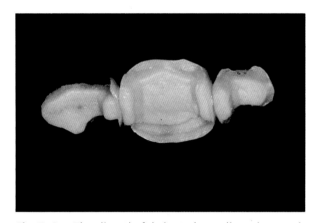

Fig 5–8 The directly fabricated, acrylic resin, provisional onlay is splinted between the two provisional inlays.

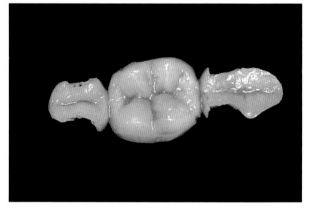

Fig 5–9 Occlusal view of the completed acrylic resin provisional restorations.

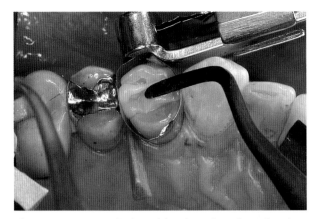

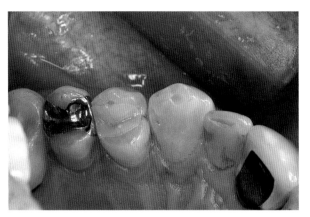

Fig 5–10 A matrix band is placed and wedged to prevent excess flow of the composite resin beyond the preparation. The composite resin is layered in incrementally, *but without the use of any bonding agent or etching.* Note color differentials to facilitate recognition during removal of the provisional restoration.

Fig 5–11 The direct composite resin provisional restoration is placed to maintain accurate tooth-to-tooth relationships.

genol-based cement (eg, Provicell, Septodont) to prevent contamination of the cavity with eugenol, which affects the subsequent curing of the composite resin luting agent. If a provisional restoration is repeatedly dislodged from the preparation between appointments, it is probably ill-fitting and may need to be relined. It is also possible, but probably inadvisable, to use a polyacrylic cement of harder consistency, such as Duralon (ESPE-Premier) which can be extremely difficult to remove from the cavity preparation.

Fortunately, patients experience little postoperative sensitivity between the preparation and seating appointments with these types of restorations because the dentin within the preparation is usually covered with a glass-ionomer base. Retention of the provisional restorations may be somewhat difficult with one or two individual units when using direct-indirect acrylic resin provisionalization, but it is seldom a problem when a quadrant of continuous provisional inlays is placed. Similarly, when an onlay or full crown is interspersed between two inlays (Fig 5–7) the provisional restoration is developed in a strip of three units joined interproximally (Figs 5–8 and 5–9). In the case of one or two individual units, use of a nonremovable direct composite resin provisional restoration is preferred.

Direct Method

Direct Composite Resin Provisional Restoration With or Without Vacuform Matrix

This is a considerably easier approach to provisionalization for individual units. There are, however, certain drawbacks to this method in that it will necessitate making the impression before provisionalization, which then negates use of the provisional restoration to measure the thickness or depth of the preparation.

After inlay preparation and subsequent impression making, the tooth is dried and coated with a very thin layer of lubricant (eg, petroleum jelly or silicone); this will prevent desiccation of the glass-ionomer base during the provisional restoration fabrication procedure. A thin, dead-soft matrix band is placed interproximally and wedged tightly to prevent overextension of the provisional restorative material into the proximal embrasure (Fig 5–10). The composite resin is now placed in the preparation in incremental sections, starting in the base of the interproximal box. The resin is placed in much the same way as it is for a conventional composite resin restoration, but without the process of enamel etching or the use of any bonding agent. The usual concerns associated with composite resin polymerization shrinkage are not a factor because this interim restoration is not bonded to the tooth; hence there are no tensile stresses on the cusps. The usual sensitivity, caused by lack of marginal integrity and an adequate seal, is seldom a problem because the dentin was previously covered by a glass-ionomer base.

The color selected for the composite resin of the provisional restoration must not be similar to the color of the tooth, so that the restoration is easily distinguished from tooth substance during removal. Once the composite resin is in position and cured, the matrix band is removed and the curing procedure is completed from the buccal and lingual surfaces.

The composite resin provisional restoration is then adjusted for lateral excursions while an accurate centric hold is maintained. The football-shaped finishing instrument (eg, E.T. O.S.I., Brasseler Corp) works ideally. Remaining excess in the interproximal region can be trimmed with the tapered 30-blade finishing carbide (eg, E.T., Brasseler Corp.), which is unlikely to inadvertently remove a preparation margin. Centric occlusion and all excursive movements of the mandible are checked once again with articulating paper.

The provisional inlay plays a critical role in maintaining the accuracy of the intra-arch and interarch relationships (Fig 5–11). Porcelain, unlike gold, cannot be readily adjusted and polished; therefore it is essential to accurately maintain the relationships present at the time of impression making.

At the seating appointment it may be necessary to section the provisional composite resin inlay for removal, despite the previous lubrication. This is the reason for using a composite resin that is a different color than the tooth, so that recognition of the composite resin within the confines of the preparation is possible. If the composite resin for any reason becomes dislodged during its fabrication, it can simply be polished before being replaced in the preparation with a non–eugenol-based cement.

At no stage during provisionalization is enamel etching done, nor is any form of bonding agent used.

Indirect Method

Indirect Composite Resin/Acrylic Resin Provisional Restorations

Indirect provisional restorations are fabricated in a laboratory on a working cast of the preparations (Fig 5–12). An impression of the preparation is made and poured in a rapidly setting die material. A vacuform matrix prepared on an original study cast or a preoperative alginate impression is filled with a soupy mix of acrylic resin. This is gently manipulated into position on the lubricated cast of the prepared teeth (Fig 5–13), held in position during the initial cure, and manipulated on and off the working cast to prevent its locking into any undercuts. The cured resin inlays are trimmed to the margins of the prepared teeth on the master cast, and the occlusal surfaces are accurately developed (Fig 5–14). The embrasure form is created between the teeth, but adjacent provisional restorations are maintained in one continuous strip. The restorations are returned to the mouth, where marginal integrity is checked and any occlusal discrepancies are adjusted. The provisional inlays are removed once again and returned to the laboratory, where final occlusal anatomy is developed and polishing and staining is completed (Figs 15a and b). They must be cemented into position with a non–eugenol-based cement and the excess cement must be carefully removed. The patient must be instructed on the use of floss threaders for cleaning interproximally when adjacent provisional restorations are joined.

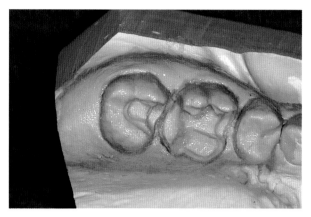

Fig 5–12   Working cast of two inlay preparations.

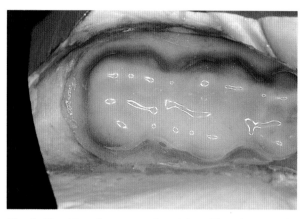

Fig 5–13   Vacuform matrix with self-curing acrylic resin in position over working cast of preparations.

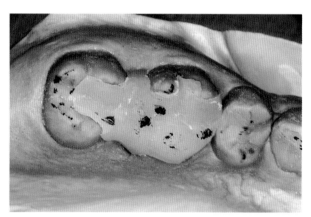

Fig 5–14   Developing occlusal relationships and marginal integrity.

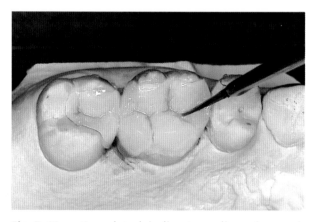

Fig 5–15a   Completed indirect acrylic resin provisional restorations, stained and characterized.

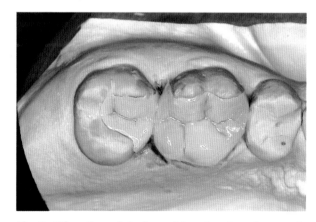

Fig 5–15b   Completed provisional restoration ready for cementation.

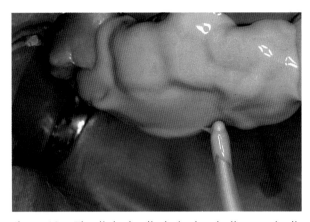

Fig 5–16 The light-bodied vinyl polysiloxane is directly syringed into the preparation and sulcus from an automix system (Reprosil, LD Caulk).

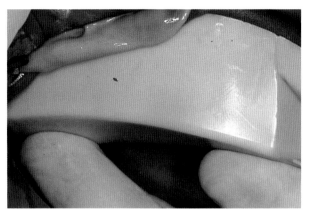

Fig 5–17 The heavy-bodied mixed putty in a stock tray displaces the light-bodied material apically and supports it accurately.

Impression Techniques

Etched porcelain inlays and onlays are generally fabricated on some form of master cast. This working cast must be an accurate reproduction of the preparation, and the impression material is selected from those commonly used for crown-and-bridge techniques. These include all the elastomeric impression materials, such as polysulfides, polyethers, condensation silicones, and vinyl polysiloxanes (addition silicones). Hydrocolloid is a slightly more complex impression material, in that it tends to tear in the unprepared undercut areas between or below the contact areas and because a refractory die material cannot be poured directly into it. This situation would then require that a secondary elastomeric impression be made of the first cast poured from the hydrocolloid in the laboratory. Hence the master cast would be a second-generation cast, which would increase the chances for inaccuracies. Hydrocolloid may also be inconvenient because of the need to pour the impression immediately within the office.

In general, when fabricating quadrants of etched porcelain inlays or onlays, ceramists find it more convenient to have two complete-arch impressions. An alternative technique for individual teeth or for small numbers of units is the dual-impression system, made using the triple tray (ESPE-Premier).

Tissue Management

The inlay preparation should end supragingivally or just within the confines of the sulcus so as not to infringe on the biologic width interproximally. For accurate impressions, it is essential that the tissues be managed with electrosurgery or be laterally displaced with astringent impregnated cords.

When multiple adjacent teeth are to be treated in the same quadrant, it is often necessary to use electrosurgery, because it is difficult to displace a papilla both mesially and distally to secure an impression of adjacent interproximal boxes.

When retraction cord is used, the cord should remain in position for about 7 minutes. It should be made wet with a water syringe before being removed, to avoid tearing of the tenuous junctional epithelium, which would create hemorrhage.

The base of the interproximal box of the preparation must not infringe on the biologic width — it should be no closer than 2 mm to the osseous crest. If the box begins to impinge on this dimension, untoward periodontal reactions are invariably the result, and prerestorative elective surgery might be preferable.

When the interproximal box is not deep, it may be possible to make impressions with the rubber dam in place.

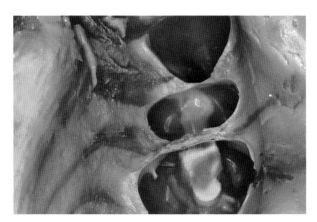

Fig 5–18 The impression is examined for surface detail, fissure lines, and voids.

Impression Making

The impression material used should be of two viscosities: heavy and light. When a polysulfide is used, the heavy-bodied material is placed in a custom-fitted tray. If a vinyl polysiloxane is selected, the mixed putty is placed in a stock tray. The light-bodied, less viscous material is syringed directly into the gingival sulcus and over the preparation (Fig 5–16). A chip syringe can be used to air blow this light-bodied material into the sulcus as well as into all angles of the preparation. The heavy-bodied material then displaces the syringed, light-bodied material into the preparation and sulcus beyond the finish line and supports it (Fig 5–17). The automixed systems for vinyl polysiloxanes make this whole process simple, accurate, and predictable. After the appropriate time, the impression material is removed and checked for surface detail, voids, and integrity of all the finish lines (Fig 5–18). The impression material is allowed to set for the appropriate time before the master cast is poured (see chapter 2). The impression material should have high tensile strength, good surface detail, and low deformation. In addition, for today's dentistry, it is essential to be able to disinfect the impression before pouring without the disinfection process causing distortions.

Shade Selection

When a shade is selected for the final ceramic restoration, it is advisable to err slightly on the lighter side. It is easier to modify toward a darker color with a composite resin luting material than it is to lighten the restoration shade with the composite resin luting agent. *In addition, the use of a lighter composite resin luting agent to compensate for dark porcelain can result in an unesthetic white line around the restoration.* Fortunately, this type of etched restoration has a certain chameleonlike effect caused by the translucent nature of the porcelain. Therefore, such restorations blend in remarkably well. The ceramist will, however, require information on such aspects as staining in the fissures, texture, degree of translucency, and other special effects.

The ceramist should also be able to mount the casts accurately, so that occlusal relations in maximum intercuspation occlusions and lateral excursions of the mandible are correctly developed in the laboratory. This should negate, or at least minimize, the amount of intraoral adjustment of the restoration. Such adjustments destroy the surface finish and the anatomic carvings, leaving a potentially more abrasive surface against the opposing teeth and reportedly dramatically increasing the wear of the opposing occlusion.

Laboratory Procedures

6

Pinhas Adar

The technique for etched porcelain inlays and onlays is, in many ways, an extension of the procedures used for etched porcelain laminate veneers. The obvious difference is that for veneers the tooth preparation is extracoronal, whereas for the etched porcelain inlay or onlay it is predominantly an intracoronal process. The immediate problem that this difference brings to the fore is that it is exceptionally difficult to use the platinum foil technique, because of the problems in adapting foil to the internal aspects of a tooth preparation and then being able to remove the foil without distortion. The refractory investment technique thus becomes a more viable alternative.

Communication with the ceramist is of the utmost importance, as porcelain inlays and onlays are invariably done predominantly for esthetic reasons. The restorations are fabricated indirectly, and quite often at a site distant from the office, so that the ceramist requires as much information on the prescription form as possible: detailed shade selection breakdown with information regarding cervical, body, and enamel colors, as well as particulars associated with specific characterizations (Fig 6–1). Visual aids, such as photographic slides and line drawings, will communicate to the technician the specific needs of the patient. Obviously, accurate impressions of the preparations and the opposing arch, as well as a bite registration, are also essential.

Refractory Investment Technique

Unlike porcelain laminate veneers, for which the platinum foil system is often the system of choice, inlays should be fabricated with the *refractory die technique.* This necessitates developing a master cast with interchangeable master dies and refractory dies, using the keyed types of interlocking trays.

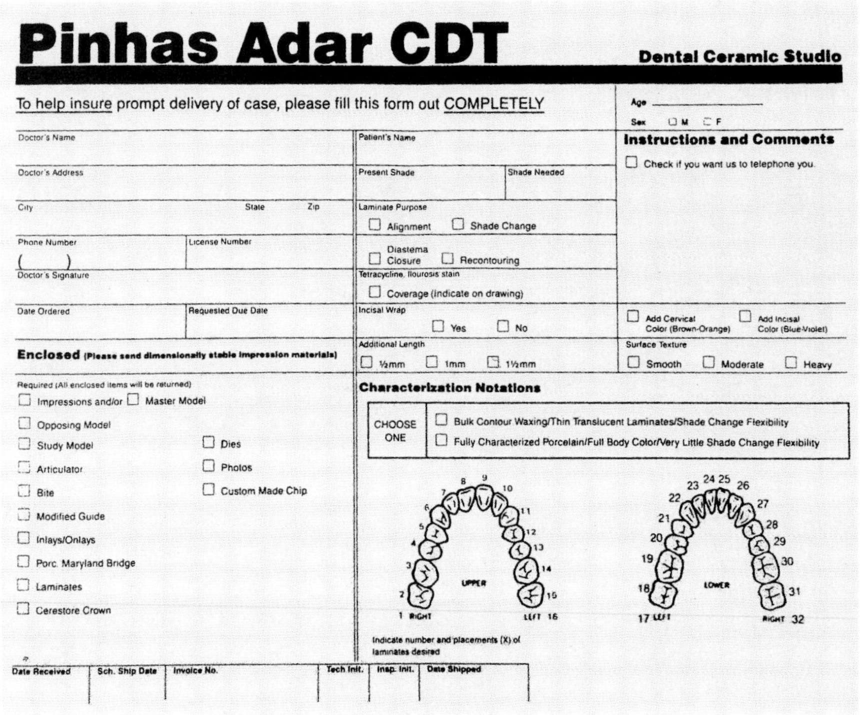

Pinhas Adar CDT

Dental Ceramic Studio

To help insure prompt delivery of case, please fill this form out COMPLETELY

Age _____
Sex ☐ M ☐ F

Doctor's Name

Patient's Name

Instructions and Comments

☐ Check if you want us to telephone you.

Doctor's Address

Present Shade | Shade Needed

City | State | Zip

Laminate Purpose
☐ Alignment ☐ Shade Change

Phone Number | License Number
(   )

☐ Diastema Closure ☐ Recontouring

Doctor's Signature

Tetracycline, flourosis stain
☐ Coverage (indicate on drawing)

Date Ordered | Requested Due Date

Incisal Wrap
☐ Yes ☐ No

☐ Add Cervical Color (Brown-Orange) ☐ Add Incisal Color (Blue-Violet)

Enclosed (Please send dimensionally stable impression materials)

Additional Length
☐ ½mm ☐ 1mm ☐ 1½mm

Surface Texture
☐ Smooth ☐ Moderate ☐ Heavy

Required (All enclosed items will be returned)
☐ Impressions and/or ☐ Master Model
☐ Opposing Model
☐ Study Model ☐ Dies
☐ Articulator ☐ Photos
☐ Bite ☐ Custom Made Chip
☐ Modified Guide
☐ Inlays/Onlays
☐ Porc. Maryland Bridge
☐ Laminates
☐ Cerestore Crown

Characterization Notations

CHOOSE ONE
☐ Bulk Contour Waxing/Thin Translucent Laminates/Shade Change Flexibility
☐ Fully Characterized Porcelain/Full Body Color/Very Little Shade Change Flexibility

Indicate number and placements (X) of laminates desired

Date Received | Sch. Ship Date | Invoice No. | Tech Init. | Insp. Init. | Date Shipped

Fig 6–1 Laboratory communication: the ceramist must be given all the necessary information to fabricate the restoration.

Developing the Master Cast

The impressions from the dentist are poured initially in a hard die stone, as for standard crown-and-bridge technique. The impression is then taken to the laboratory where it is disinfected prior to the pouring process. The internal aspect of the impression is treated with a surface tension–reducing solution to facilitate pouring without the development of voids and distortions.

The die stone is poured into the impression to about *1 inch beyond the free gingival margin* (Fig 6–2) and allowed to bench set for at least 30 minutes. When the die stone is completely set, the cast is released from the impression and cut back on a cast trimmer, creating a flat surface for the base. This base surface should remain at least 1 cm from the free gingival margin so that during the "pindexing" process, the base of the pin does not encroach the preparations on the die.

A reliable pinning system is used to individually pin all the teeth to be restored (Fig 6–3). The adjacent teeth are pinned as a single unit or in large convenient sections. Because accuracy is of paramount importance, the double-pinning technique is recommended.

The pin-indexed master cast is lubricated with a separating medium, and a base of yellow stone is poured onto this around the dowel pins. This process localizes the individual sections accurately and predictably. The entire complex is allowed to harden before it is trimmed and separated into the component parts (Fig 6–4). The completed master cast is lifted off the newly formed base, and the individual dies are sectioned from it by cutting from the bottom to the gingival area interproximally. Sections are then gently snapped apart at this friable junction to maintain accuracy. The sectioning into individual dies is easily accomplished with a jeweler's saw or a rotary diamond disk on a laboratory handpiece.

The individual dies are trimmed to reduce the amount of die stem material surrounding the dowel pins; this allows easier handling and replacement onto the base (Fig 6–5).

Developing the Master Cast (Figs 6–2 to 6–9)

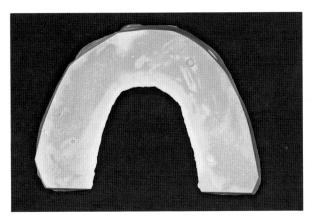

Fig 6–2 The impression has been poured about 1 inch beyond the free gingival margin and is here shown prior to pin-indexing and the second pour for the base.

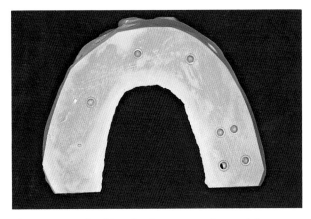

Fig 6–3 A double-pinning system is used for accurate localization of the individual dies on the working cast.

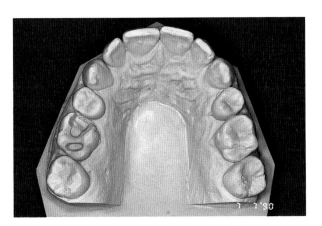

Fig 6–4 Completed master cast comprising the individual dies and the base.

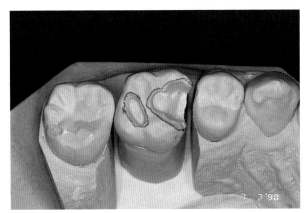

Fig 6–5 Individual trimmed die with the reduced die stem shown on the master cast.

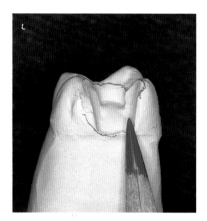

Fig 6–6 The marginal periphery of the preparation is outlined with a red lead pencil.

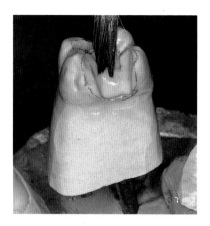

Fig 6–7 The die is sealed with a light-cured resin.

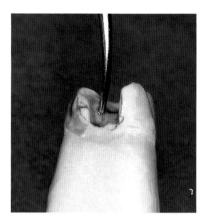

Fig 6–8 The internal fitting surface of the preparation is treated with an oil-based red wax, which effectively acts as a die spacer.

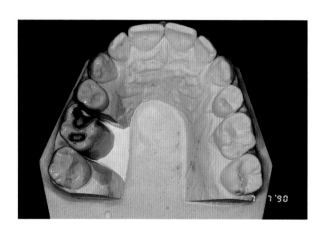

Fig 6–9 Reassembled master cast ready for duplication of the dies.

The interproximal margins in Class II or compound preparations are carefully ditched to the margins. It is important to reduce the amount of extraneous material on these individual dies so that when the refractory die is made it is of the most minimal size. This reduces the available amount of refractory material left to retain heat during the fabrication process.

The margins are outlined on the die with a red lead pencil (Fig 6–6), and the die is sealed with a light-cured resin (Fig 6–7). The individual dies

are surveyed to ascertain whether there are any undercuts or imperfections.

The internal fitting surface of the preparation is treated with an oil-based red wax, which acts as a die spacer (Fig 6–8). The benefit of the wax, as compared to conventional die spacer, is that when the final restoration is retrofitted on the master cast, the wax die spacing can be readily removed with boiling water. The master cast is now reassembled and ready for duplication of the dies in refractory material (Fig 6–9).

Generating the Refractory Dies

The choice of phosphate-bonded refractory investment material should be based on the coefficient of thermal expansion of the ceramic system being used to fabricate the restoration. If the coefficients of thermal expansion of the die material and ceramic are too different, inaccuracies and distortions will occur and the restoration will not fit.

There are several different systems for duplicating the working cast. A relatively simple technique, especially for multiple units, uses the Modi-Vet System (Jeneric/Pentron). In this system the working cast is placed on a flat metallic base with a plastic liner above it. The entire cast is covered with a clear mold containing several large holes in its top surface (Fig 6–10); it is held in position with three magnets. A vinyl polysiloxane material (Fig 6–11) is mixed according to the manufacturer's instructions and slowly poured through one of the holes in the mold's top (Fig 6–12). The material should spread slowly, encompassing the cast, while avoiding the incorporation of air bubbles or voids. This material is allowed to set (Fig 6–13) according to the specific instructions of the manufacturer.

When the plate is separated from the mold, the vinyl polysiloxane remains in the mold and is incorporated in the working cast (Fig 6–14). The yellow stone base is removed (Fig 6–15), leaving only the tooth portions of the master cast located in the vinyl polysiloxane. Now the specific individual dies of the preparations are removed from the vinyl polysiloxane (Fig 6–16), leaving the rest of the areas in place. Only the specific preparation die regions of the vinyl polysiloxane

mold will then be repoured in the refractory investment material (Fig 6–17). Special heat-resistant pins (Thermo-Pins I and II, New Generation Restorations, Jeneric/Pentron) (Fig 6–18) are placed in the newly poured dies of refraction investment (Fig 6–19). It is important to ensure that these new pins are placed parallel to the previous double pins of the rest of the cast; if they are divergent, the base will not separate from the working cast.

Once the refractory investment is set, the entire new working cast is lubricated with a separating medium (Fig 6–20). The refractory die material seems to be best lubricated with a thin layer of petroleum jelly. A thin strip of orthodontic wax is placed on the ends of the pins and a small ball of wax is placed on the end of the refractory die, so they can be readily found once a new base is poured. The new base is poured to occupy the remaining space in the master mold and allowed to set once again (Fig 6–21). Now the actual working cast with the dies in the exact same relationship as on the master cast is separated, and the refractory dies will be located precisely and accurately (Fig 6–22). This process of separation from the refractory die must be done by peeling the impression away from the refractory, because simply pulling it out will result in loss of surface detail. (When necessary, this entire cast can be articulated on whatever particular system the technician prefers.)

This base is trimmed on a cast trimmer until the wax shows through. The wax is removed, leaving the ends of the pins clearly evident (Fig 6–23). Pushing on the base of the pin will pop the individual die loose, and the die is then ready to be worked on.

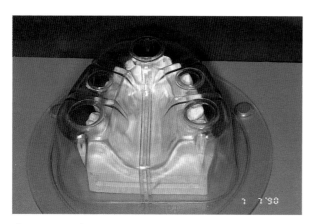

Fig 6–10   The entire master cast is covered with a clear mold that contains several large holes in its top surface and is attached to the underlying base with three magnets.

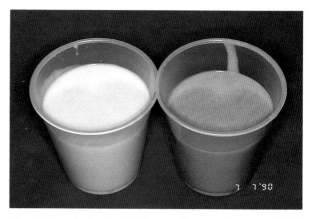

Fig 6–11   A vinyl polysiloxane impression material is mixed according to the manufacturer's instructions.

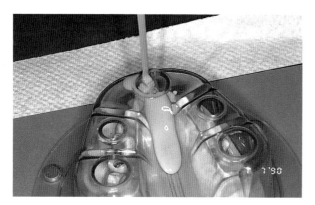

Fig 6–12   The impression material is poured slowly through one of the three large holes in the top of the mold and allowed to slowly spread and encompass the entire cast.

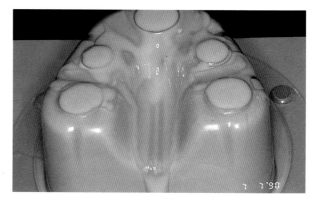

Fig 6–13   Completed refractory impression in the mold.

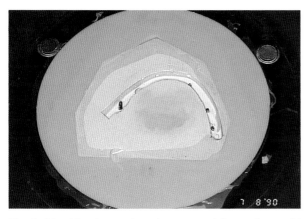

Fig 6–14 The base plate is removed from the mold with the impression, which incorporates the working cast.

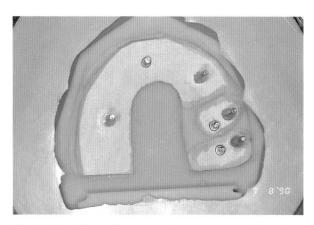

Fig 6–15 The yellow stone base is removed, leaving the tooth aspect of the master cast firmly located in the vinyl polysiloxane impression material.

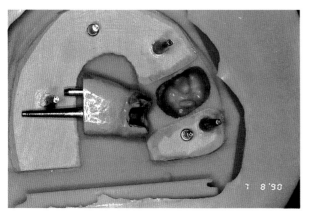

Fig 6–16 The die of the prepared tooth or teeth is removed from the impression material.

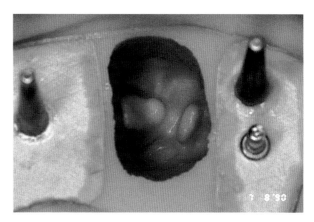

Fig 6–17 This specific portion of the impression will be repoured in a refractory investment.

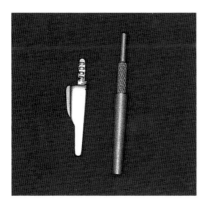

Fig 6–18 Heat-resistant pinning system for the refractory die.

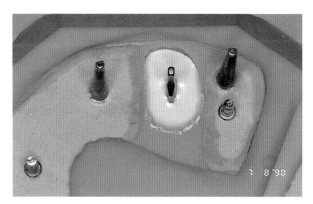

Fig 6–19 The impression is poured in a refractory investment and repinned parallel to the original pins in the rest of the cast.

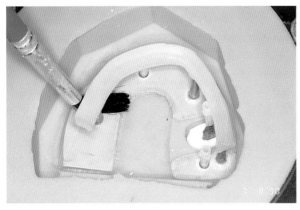

Fig 6–20 The tooth portions are again lubricated with a separating medium, and the ends of the pins are covered with a thin strip of orthodontic wax.

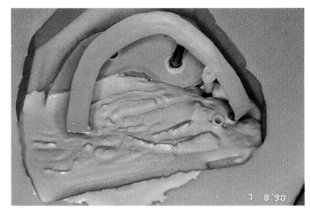

Fig 6–21 A new yellow stone base is poured.

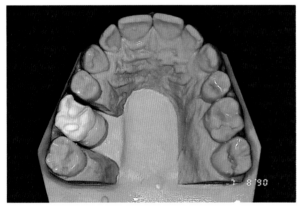

Fig 6–22 The die or dies on the working cast should have exactly the same relationship as they do on the original master cast.

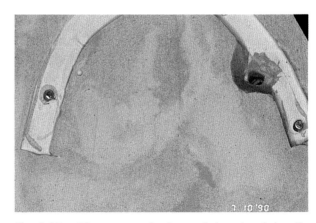

Fig 6–23 The wax on the base of the pin of the die begins to show through as the base of the new working cast is trimmed. Once this wax is removed, the ends of the pins are easy to pop out of the base.

Porcelain Buildup

The refractory dies are marked; ie, the periphery or finish line of the preparation is outlined with a specially formulated refractory marker (Fig 6–24) that will be incorporated into the refractory material following degassing. The refractory dies are degassed according to the specific manufacturer's instructions (Fig 6–25). This removes organic contaminants and starts to fuse the ceramic binders in the die material.

After the refractory dies have been removed from the furnace and allowed to cool, they are soaked in distilled water before the porcelain buildup is begun (Fig 6–26). Before each application of porcelain, and following the previous bake, the dies must once again be cooled and then soaked in distilled water for a minimum of 1 minute, until the bubbles stop appearing and the investment material has imbibed all the water it can.

There are several different methods of sealing the refractory material before the actual porcelain buildup. The technique described is efficacious, but it is not the only option.

Preparing for Porcelain Buildup (Figs 6–24 to 6–26)

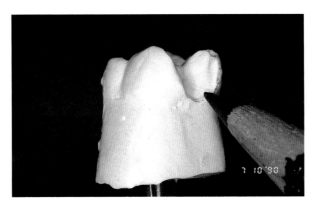

Fig 6–24   The refractory die is marked with a blue, specially formulated refractory marker, so that the marginal periphery of the restoration is delineated.

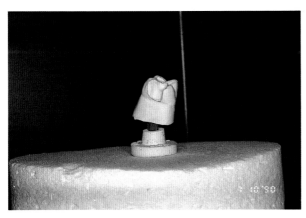

Fig 6–25   Degassing process of the refractory die.

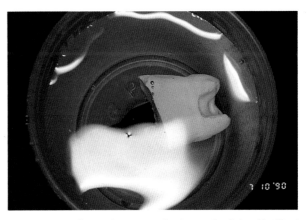

Fig 6–26   The refractory die is soaked in distilled water prior to porcelain buildup.

Sealing the Refractory Die

The marginal areas and the most lateral aspects of the walls of the cavity are covered with a very thin layer of a translucent porcelain mix (Fig 6–27). This acts as a sealing layer.

Base Layers

The base or pulpal aspect of the cavity is covered with a fine mix of opacious dentin or core mate- rial of relatively higher chroma. This thin layer of porcelain is baked according to the manufacturer's recommended firing cycles (Fig 6–28). Once this has come out of the furnace and been allowed to cool fully, the entire die is soaked again in distilled water for about 2 minutes (Fig 6–29). This can be followed by layering a veneer of translucent porcelain on the marginal areas to facilitate a blending-in of the color of the final restorations.

Sealing and Base Layers (Figs 6–27 to 6–29)

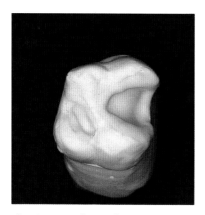

Fig 6–27 The refractory die is sealed. A thin layer of translucent porcelain mix is adapted to the marginal areas and the lateral aspects of the cavity preparation to act as a sealing layer.

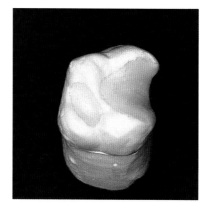

Fig 6–28 The base or pulpal aspect of the cavity is covered with a thin mix of opacious dentin or core material of relatively high chroma.

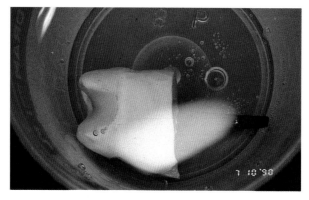

Fig 6–29 Once this initial bake has cooled, the entire die is soaked in the distilled water again for about 2 minutes.

Body Buildup

Depending on the size of the restoration, the subsequent ceramic layers are built up incrementally. This incremental approach allows for sintering shrinkage to be continually compensated for, thereby decreasing the potential for marginal discrepancies. *In general, more and smaller incremental bakes result in fewer potential fractures and marginal discrepancies.* The dentin buildup (Fig 6–30) occupies the deeper aspects of the cavity preparation and is completed before the superficial enamel layers are finished. If very thick, these layers can be split down the central fossa to allow for shrinkage toward the walls during firing.

The final surface of about 0.5 mm is built up in a more translucent porcelain enamel (Fig 6–31) to restore complete form and anatomic detail to the tooth. An endodontic finger spreader or similar instrument can be used to develop a line of cleavage down the central fossa. When fired, the porcelain will shrink toward the area of greatest bulk against the walls of the cavity,

opening up this cleavage slightly. The cuspal inclinations and primary and secondary anatomy are similarly developed, and the interproximal box form is restored (Fig 6–32).

Once the final bake is completed, the contacts are marked (Fig 6–33) and adjusted (Fig 6–34) with a fine diamond rotary instrument to fit the master cast. The occlusal relations are checked and adjusted for maximum intercuspation or centric occlusion and lateral excursive movements of the mandible (Fig 6–35).

Final shaping is completed with rotary diamond points and fine carbide burs (Fig 6–36). Excess porcelain beyond the marked margin (refractory material and overextended porcelain) is trimmed away with a rotary diamond disk (Fig 6–37). The finish line should be delineated accurately, but the restoration margin may not be totally cut back at this stage. The margins will be finished just before the rest of the refractory investment is sandblasted away, after staining and glazing.

Body Buildup (Figs 6–30 to 6–37)

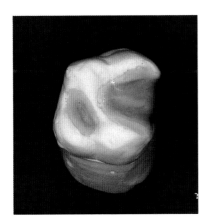

Fig 6–30 The dentin buildup is completed within the deep aspects of the cavity preparation before the final enamel layers are added.

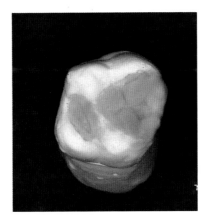

Fig 6–31 A surface layer of about 0.5 mm is built up in translucent porcelain enamel to restore complete form and anatomic detail to the tooth.

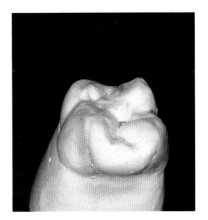

Fig 6–32 The secondary anatomy and interproximal aspects of the compound cavity are completed.

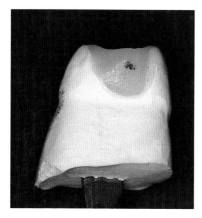

Fig 6–33 The contacts are marked with articulating paper.

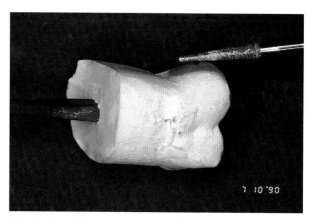

Fig 6–34 After the porcelain has baked and cooled, the contacts are marked to allow for complete seating on the master cast. If the contacts are tight, they are adjusted with a fine diamond rotary instrument.

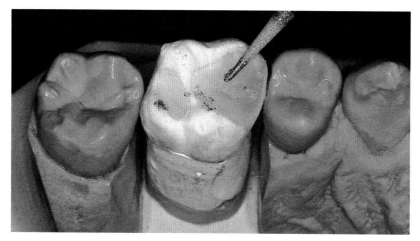

Fig 6–35 The occlusion is adjusted for both maximum intercuspation and excursive mandibular movements.

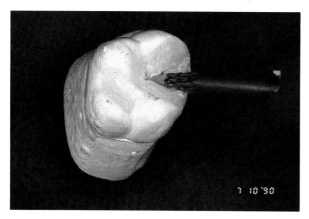

Fig 6–36 The final form is completed with rotary diamond points and fine carbide burs.

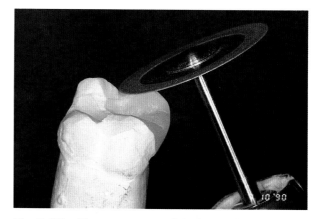

Fig 6–37 The excess porcelain beyond the marked margin is trimmed with a rotary diamond disk.

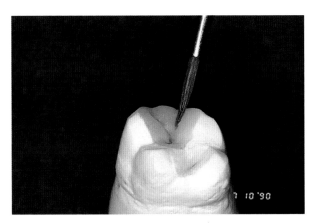

Fig 6–38   A thin layer of glaze and any characterizing stain are applied to the completed restoration.

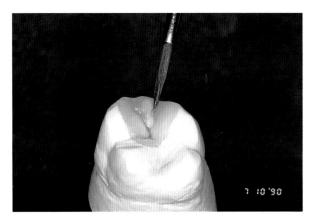

Fig 6–39   The cast is highlighted with a milky white stain.

Staining and Glazing

Once anatomic detail and the margins are almost completed, the die and restoration are soaked once again in distilled water. A thin layer of glaze and any stain porcelains are applied over the restoration surface (Fig 6–38). The separation created by the endodontic finger spreader facilitates easy placement of the stain in the central and lateral fossae. The cusp tips may be highlighted with a milky white stain, and any specific individualized characterization is added (Fig 6–39). The restoration is now heated in the furnace to the desired temperature and allowed to cool.

Releasing the Restoration—Fitting and Finishing

Once the restoration has cooled, the remaining refractory investment is blasted away with glass beads (Fig 6–40). These beads should not damage the porcelain but will remove the investment. The released restoration is retrofitted to the original stone master cast, from which the die-spacing wax has been removed by steam cleaning or soaking in boiling water (Fig 6–41).

The restorations are placed individually on the original stone dies of the master cast (Fig 6–42), and any excess porcelain flash remaining from the original margin delineation is now gently abraded with a fine gray porcelain-finishing wheel (Fig 6–43).

The marginal integrity of each restoration is developed on this cast. The contact relationships are adjusted on a third cast, which has been poured but never sectioned, so that contacts remain absolutely accurate (Fig 6–44).

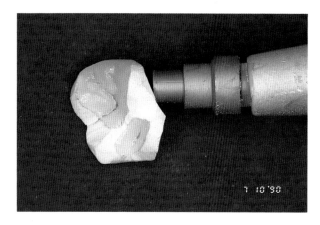

Fig 6–40 The remaining refractory investment is removed with glass beads in a sandblaster.

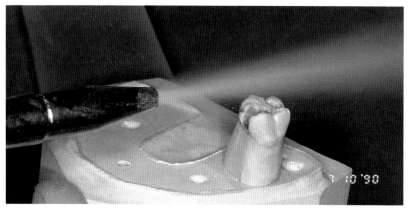

Fig 6–41 The die-spacing wax is removed from the original master cast with steam.

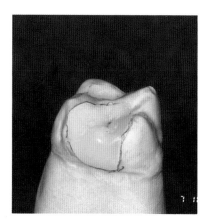

Fig 6–42 The restorations are retrofitted to the original stone dies of the master cast.

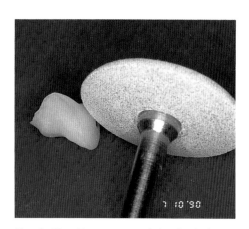

Fig 6–43 Excess porcelain flash is removed with a fine-grained porcelain finishing wheel.

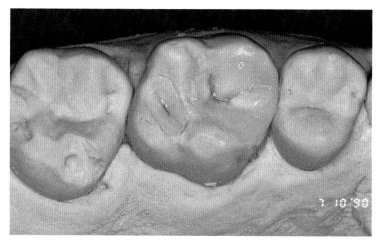

Fig 6–44 Final adjustments of contacts are made on the third (nonsectioned) cast.

Etching

The etching process requires that the occlusal surface be covered with a layer of wax (Fig 6–45). This is because, unlike laminates, inlays have fitting surfaces with several different aspects, and the etching acid may be brushed over onto the occlusal surface. The wax therefore protects against acidic damage. The acid is squeezed out of the bottle (eg, Super Etch Mirage, Chameleon Dental) and allowed to remain on the fitting surface for 90 seconds (Fig 6–46). Once this is completed, the inlay is cleaned in the ultrasonic unit in denatured alcohol and then etched by using one of the commercial hydrofluoric acid techniques. The restorations are then ready to be luted in place (Fig 6–47).

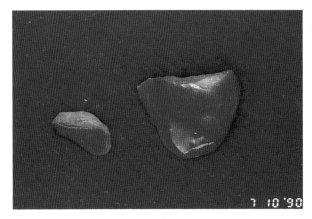

Fig 6–45   The occlusal surface is covered with a layer of wax to protect it from the acid.

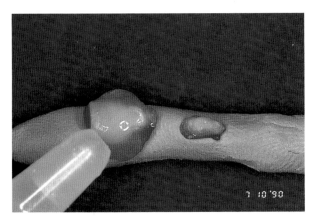

Fig 6–46   The fitting surfaces of the ceramic restorations are etched.

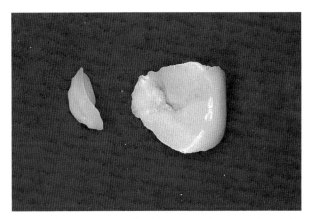

Fig 6–47   Two completed restorations ready to be luted in position.

Placement Procedures

7

Evaluating the Porcelain Restoration

Once an existing amalgam restoration (Fig 7–1) has been removed, the compromised tooth is prepared (Fig 7–2) and an impression is made and sent to the laboratory. The porcelain restorations will be returned from the laboratory with the fitting or internal surface etched and, in some instances, presilanated (Fig 7–3). Prior to the placement procedure, the porcelain restorations should be tried in the patient's mouth and assessed for four different aspects: *(1)* marginal fit and interproximal contact relations, *(2)* occlusion, *(3)* etching, and *(4)* contamination.

Marginal Fit and Interproximal Contacts

Each restoration must be checked on the master cast for intimacy of fit (Fig 7–4). Although the inlays will be placed with a composite resin luting material and not a conventional cement,

there should only be a nominal tolerance of marginal discrepancy. The margins should be closed to the greatest possible degree and in the same plane as the adjacent enamel; that is, there should be a continuation of the coronal and cuspal profile of the tooth (Fig 7–5).

The porcelain should neither extend beyond the prepared enamel surface nor be short of it. This is obviously most critical in the gingival margin area at the base of any interproximal box preparation (Fig 7–5), which is difficult to adjust once the inlay is luted in position. Any lateral overextension of porcelain in the interproximal box region can be evaluated on the master cast with a sharp explorer and unwaxed dental floss. If there is an overextension laterally into this interproximal area it must be adjusted before the restoration is luted in place. This can be done chairside with a microfine finishing diamond (eg, E.T. Series, Brasseler Corp), and the porcelain can be gently machined until it is confluent with the die. An explorer should pass over the porcelain-die junction relatively imperceptibly and should remain in the same plane as it traverses from the die (representative of the tooth surface) onto the porcelain restoration. The mar-

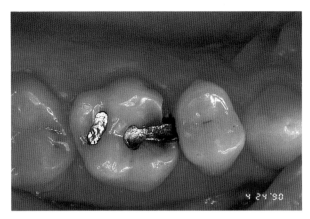

Fig 7–1 Preoperative occlusal view of failing mesio-occlusal amalgam restoration with separate occlusal amalgam restoration in the distal fossa of the maxillary molar.

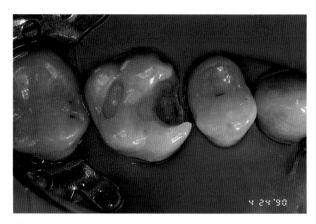

Fig 7–2 Preparation of compound mesio-occlusal inlay cavity and occlusal preparation in the distal fossa.

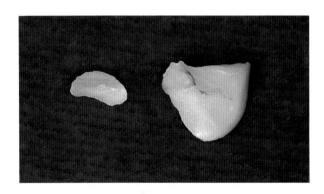

Fig 7–3 The occlusal and fitting surfaces of the two inlays as returned from the ceramic laboratory.

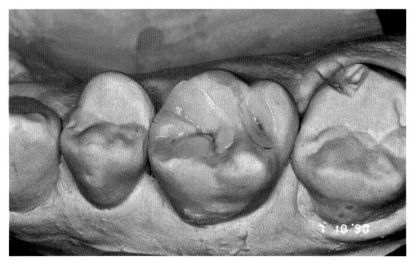

Fig 7–4 The fit of the etched ceramic restoration on the master cast is assessed.

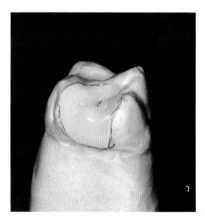

Fig 7–5 Interproximal view of etched ceramic restoration on master cast. Intimacy of fit and ceramic overhang, as well as occlusal cuspal profile, are evaluated.

gins of the restoration should all be checked to ensure that they are smooth and contiguous and have no overhangs or fractures.

If multiple restorations are to be seated, they should all be seated on the master cast together and checked for interproximal contact relationships in both buccolingual and occlusoapical dimensions. The form of each porcelain interproximal surface should be a mirror image of the adjacent tooth, and the contact should be tight enough to prevent dental floss from slipping through too easily.

Occlusion

When multiple units are to be fabricated, it is advisable to make a full-arch impression of the preparations so that the master cast can be accurately articulated with an opposing cast. This will enhance visualization of centric holding areas and all working and nonworking movements. The full-arch impression is critical for etched porcelain restorations because it is extremely difficult to adjust these friable, tiny porcelain pieces for occlusal discrepancies before the restorations are bonded to the tooth. The fracture potential at this stage demands precision and accuracy in the laboratory phase of fabrication. If the clinician is forced to remove large amounts of porcelain occlusally once the restoration is bonded in position, the intrinsic beauty and esthetic factors will be severely compromised. Also, large amounts of time will then be required to refinish and polish the porcelain to diminish its abrasive surface so as not to cause wear on the opposing arch.

To facilitate precise laboratory fabrication, every possible aid should be included with the laboratory prescription. The fabricated restorations should be checked for contact relations in centric occlusion as well as excursive movements of the mandible. This will be most critical in onlay restorations, where sufficient clearance must be developed in any lateral movements to prevent working and nonworking interferences.

The preparation must facilitate the placement of a sufficiently thick layer of porcelain (at least 1.75 mm) over the cusp to be onlaid. An occlusal clearance jig is useful for checking this clearance prior to impression making.

Occlusal contacts on these restorations should be limited wherever possible to centric holding stops with immediate disarticulation in the very first millimeter of mandibular excursive movement. This lack of contact on the porcelain cuspal inclines during lateral movement will decrease the potential for wear of the opposing arch.

Etched Surface

The internal aspect of the restoration must be visibly etched. This etched surface can even be seen (although not really evaluated) with the naked eye as a somewhat opaque and frosted surface. It is important to ensure that the etching extends to the actual margin of the restoration, where an effective seal is so critical. The fitting surfaces of an inlay are somewhat more difficult to etch than is the single concave surface of a porcelain laminate veneer and require that the laboratory technician repeatedly brush the etching gel or solution to the periphery of the restoration. The actual quality of the etched surface is extremely difficult to gauge without the use of a scanning electron microscope or high-powered stereomicroscope. However, if there are any areas that appear to be shiny instead of frosty, the restoration should be returned to the laboratory for further etching. If only a tiny area is unetched, the etching can readily be done chairside with one of the newer porcelain-etching products designed for clinical use (eg, Porcelain Etch, Bisco, Inc; Ceram-etch, Gresco Products, Inc; Porce-etch, Den-Mat Corp). The specific manufacturer's instructions need to be followed for each type of material.

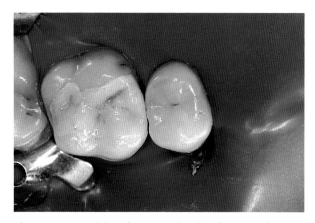

Fig 7-6 Provisional restoration in place on the prepared tooth prior to its removal for placement of the inlay.

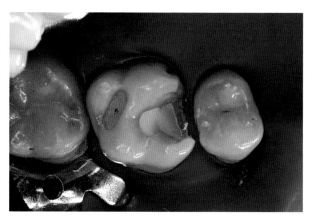

Fig 7-7 Rubber dam isolation of the preparation prevents moisture contamination during placement of the etched porcelain restoration and improves access and visualization.

Surface Contaminants, Porcelain Inclusions, and Fracture Lines

The process of fabricating small pieces of porcelain is complex and allows the tiny amounts of unfired porcelain powders to dry out fairly rapidly. If this drying out is allowed to happen before the firing, internal stresses and craze lines may develop. Once the restoration is etched, these imperfections are not readily seen and only become evident during placement, when the minor force of placing the restoration into the preparation potentiates a crack. This may also occur during polymerization shrinkage of an excessively thick layer of luting agent, which can turn a microcrack into a fracture of the restoration. The restoration should be transilluminated to check for any inclusion bodies and internal craze or crack lines.

Removal of the Provisional Restoration

The provisional restoration that was placed at the preparation and impression appointment must be removed (Fig 7-6). If this restoration was a series of acrylic resin provisional restorations joined together, it can be readily removed with either a sharp-ended, reverse-action hammer in the interproximal areas, a surgical towel clamp, or a Baade pliers. These provisional restorations are generally easier to remove than most full-coverage provisional restorations because the non–eugenol-based cements tend to be less adhesive than conventional temporary cements.

If the provisional restorations were the direct composite resin type, these can sometimes be levered out with a composite resin–removal instrument (CRNT 12, NovaTech Series, Hu-Friedy) in the interproximal contact areas and at the interface of the tooth and composite resin on the occlusal surface. It is important that the direct composite resin provisional restoration be a considerably different color than the tooth itself, so that it is readily discernible against the remaining enamel.

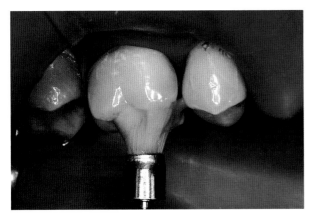

Fig 7–8   The preparation is debrided with a wet slurry of fine flour pumice and water on a small rotary bristle brush.

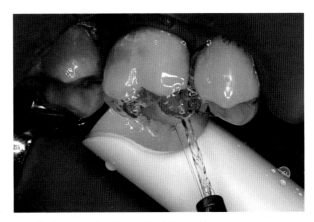

Fig 7–9   Pumice is washed from the preparation.

When it is levered out, there should be bracing for the instrument on a substantial, well-supported area of tooth that will not fracture. If the provisional restoration is not easily removable, do not force it, as this may result in problems ranging from marginal enamel chipping or fracture to complete cuspal breakage.

It is sometimes useful to bury the head of a no. 2 round bur in the occlusal surface and use it to pull out the provisional inlay. Alternatively, a no. 700 carbide bur or similarly shaped diamond can be used to section the composite resin provisional restoration before each portion of the restoration is levered out. This further emphasizes why it is so critical that the provisional restoration be a color easily distinguishable from the tooth. This allows the operator to discern the lateral periphery of the provisional restoration when sectioning it. It is important not to extend this channel laterally or apically into the tooth surface itself or into any glass-ionomer base.

With direct composite resin provisional restorations there will be no further temporary cement to remove. In the case of the indirect acrylic resin provisional restorations, any remaining temporary cementing medium must be picked out of the tooth preparation.

Rubber Dam Placement

Whenever possible, etched porcelain restorations are best luted in position under a rubber dam (Fig 7–7). The dam controls moisture contamination during this technique-sensitive stage. It also facilitates placement, provides better accessibility, and prevents accidental loss or swallowing of the restoration.

Debridement

Depending on the size and depth of the preparation, local anesthesia may be required. The prepared tooth is cleaned with a wet slurry of fine flour of pumice and water (Fig 7–8). (Use of prophylaxis pastes containing various oils and/or fluorides is generally not advocated.) This slurry is used with a small rotary prophylaxis brush to ensure that all the internal aspects of the preparation are reached. It is important to avoid injuring the interdental tissues, which may cause hemorrhaging and subsequent contamination of the etched tooth surface. The same rotary brush is used with a stream of water to remove all remnants of the pumice. The cavity is then flushed with water (Fig 7–9) and dried with an air syringe.

The Four-Stage Try-In

Prior to final luting of the porcelain inlays, it is important to follow the four-stage try-in. The restorations need to be evaluated for the following criteria:

- **Marginal integrity.** The intimate adaptation of all porcelain margins to the prepared tooth surface must be checked.
- **Proximal relations.** The collective fit and relationship of one restoration to the other or the adjacent tooth must be evaluated, as described, on the master cast.
- **Occlusal relations.** The contact relations, with the opposing arch in centric occlusion and lateral excursive movements of the mandible, *are best evaluated after inlay placement.*
- **Color.** Although these are posterior restorations, their basic shade should blend with the surrounding teeth. The need for individual characterization, such as fissure staining or other such color highlights, must also be ascertained.

The most anterior restoration is selected from the master cast and gently fitted into the respective tooth (Fig 7–10). If the restoration does not fit into position immediately, force should *not* be used. Remaining bits of the provisional restoration in the preparations or undercuts, or impingement of the contact points, should be identified and removed. If the contact needs to be adjusted, a microfine finishing diamond (E.T. Series, yellow band Brasseler Corp) can be used under magnification. Once the inlay is fitted correctly, the adjusted contact-point porcelain is finished with a series of sequential porcelain polishing points (eg, Porcelain Laminate Polishing Kit, Shofu). If there is an adjacent amalgam or similar restoration, it may be easier to adjust it, as it will polish more easily. The contact is adjusted until the restoration seats. The contact area is checked with unwaxed dental floss used in an occlusoapical direction (Fig 7–11). The floss should also be drawn upward apico-occlusally to check that there is no lateral overhang of porcelain in the interproximal gingival marginal area of the box. If necessary, this porcelain overhang should be adjusted accordingly, using the master cast as a guide. The occlusal aspect is similarly checked for marginal integrity. The remainder of the restoration is evaluated for intimacy of fit with a fine-tipped explorer (Fig 7–12).

The restoration should now also be checked for color. A harmonious shade blend is usually all that is necessary as color is considerably less critical in posterior restorations than in anterior porcelain laminate veneers. However, do not allow the teeth to dry out while they are under the rubber dam, as that will make color evaluation impossible.

The final color of the luted restoration, much like that of porcelain laminate veneers, is the result of several factors, not just the porcelain shade selected. These factors are:

1. The original tooth color
2. The porcelain shade selected and the amount of opacifier and/or translucency within the porcelain
3. The color and opacity of the composite resin luting agent

These three factors have varying influence on the final color of the luted restoration. In an anterior porcelain veneer, where the porcelain thickness is only 0.5 mm, the color is readily modified by the luting resin. In a thicker posterior restoration, the color of the porcelain is the preeminent factor and is not easily changed with the underlying resin. However, there is still an esthetic need for this porcelain restoration to blend relatively imperceptibly into the adjacent tooth structure at the junction of the restoration and the tooth preparation.

To facilitate this, the ceramist must add increasing amounts of translucent porcelain to the buildup in these peripheral areas to allow for color transference.

This, combined with the use of a more translucent composite resin luting agent, facilitates the reflectance of tooth color through the composite resin and the somewhat translucent porcelain, resulting in an imperceptible junction.

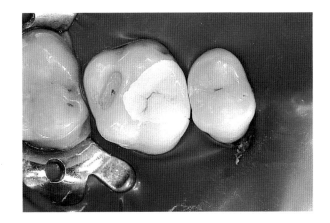

Fig 7–10 The mesio-occlusal porcelain inlay is tried in.

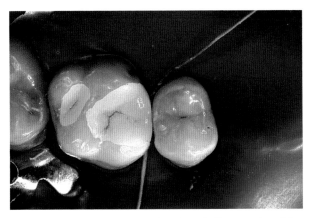

Fig 7–11 Both mesio-occlusal and disto-occlusal inlays are tried in. Proximal contact relations and any ceramic overhang are checked for with floss.

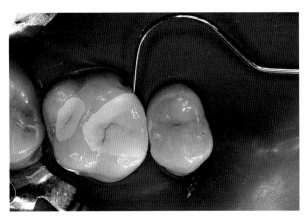

Fig 7–12 A sharp explorer is used to evaluate all peripheral margins for intimacy of fit.

During the try-in, the air refraction space between the restoration and the tooth makes it difficult to assess the actual blend in color between tooth and restoration; a light-transmitting medium is therefore required. Although products such as K-Y Lubricating Jelly (Johnson & Johnson), glycerine, or even water can be used as a trial medium, the authors prefer to use the actual luting resin or a matching trial paste of nonsetting composite resin luting agent (eg, Advanced Porcelain Restoration Kit, Den-Mat Corp; Choice, Bisco, Inc; P.V.S., Jelenko; Insure, Cosmedent; Dicor Try-In Paste, Dentsply International).

The ultimate color of the restoration will become evident once it is placed in position with this luting agent or trial paste in the interface. In general it is considerably easier to use a composite resin luting agent shade that is matched to the porcelain shade guide used (eg, Vita-Lumin, Vident; Bioform, Dentsply International). There is then a specific and direct correlation between the porcelain shade selected for the restoration itself and the composite resin luting agent, allowing the best possible blend to be achieved. Time is therefore not wasted at the try-in stage by going through noncorrelating shades of composite resin luting agents. A semitranslucent type of resin is preferable, because the more opaque the luting agent, the more likely it will show up in the interface of tooth and restoration and the less will be the transmission of color from tooth to porcelain.

In anterior laminates and inlays, such as a Class IV restoration replacing an incisal edge and covering a portion of the labial surface, this color blend is more critical. The same applies to the Class III restoration done from the labial surface, or the cervical Class V restoration, where several colors of composite resins may have to be tried to achieve an ideal blend.

In posterior restorations where the porcelain is invariably a millimeter and a half or more thick, it is important that the porcelain shade selected approximate that of the tooth, because successful modification with the composite resin luting agent is unlikely.

If the actual composite resin is used during this try-in process, the restoration and luting agent should not be exposed to the operating light for any extended period of time, as they may initiate the curing process.

It is essential to lute all restorations with a dual-cure composite resin, in which the curing process is initiated by white light and continues via a chemical-cure process (eg, Resiment, Septodont; Advanced Porcelain Restoration Kit, DenMat Corp; Choice, Bisco, Inc; Dual, Vivadent; Mirage Dual Cure, Chameleon Dental Products; Porcelite Dual Cure, Kerr/Sybron; P.V.S., Jelenko).

In those posterior restorations where exact matching is important, certain specific characterizations may be required, such as stain within the occlusal fissures or small areas of hypocalcification. If these have not been built in by the laboratory during the fabrication process, the restorations can be characterized externally with a low-fusing porcelain veneer tinting system, or the restoration can be supported with one of the rapidly setting instant investments (eg, Gresco Products), which will allow the use of conventional porcelain stains and subsequent firing while it decreases the risk that the restoration will be deformed.

Once the restoration has undergone the four-stage try-in for (1) individual fit and marginal integrity, (2) collective fit and interproximal relations, (3) occlusal relationships, and (4) color, the porcelain inlay may be removed from the tooth and placed in an ultrasonic cleaner in a container of denatured alcohol or acetone for 6 minutes. This will remove all residue of the try-in composite resin or any other contaminants. The inlay is then rinsed with water and dried.

Composite Resin Luting Agents

Several factors must be considered when the luting agent is selected.

Film Thickness

The finer the particle size in the filler, the thinner the film thickness of the luting agent. A microfill resin would therefore be ideal from this point of view. However, the microfill resin has other properties that are not as desirable.

Wear Resistance

This factor appears to be extremely important in the case of porcelain inlays, as ditching of the luting agent appears to occur at the margins over time. To decrease this, it is best to use a hybrid composite resin with a soft, small-particled glass (such as barium or strontium, rather than quartz), which appears to be more resistant to wear. In addition, the hybrid resin should be optimized; that is, the maximum potential filler should approach *70% fill as determined by volume and not by weight.* This would minimize the amount of available resin to break down at this critical junction.

Marginal Sealer and Stain Resistance

This factor is also related to the strength of the composite resin and the amount of filler it contains. A hybrid resin would suit this factor best, as it has the highest potential degree of fill and good tensile and compressive strengths.

Dual-Cure Capacity

The process of light curing allows the clinician time and flexibility during inlay placement, but curing must continue via a chemical process so that even within the deeper regions of the cavity preparation the composite resin will set.

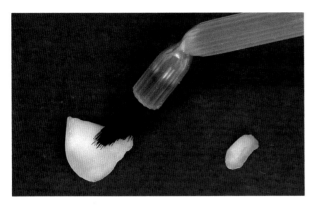

Fig 7–13 The fitting surface of the inlay is coated with a layer of silane and allowed to volatilize and dry. Color-coordinated brushes should be used to avoid confusion (eg, yellow for silane).

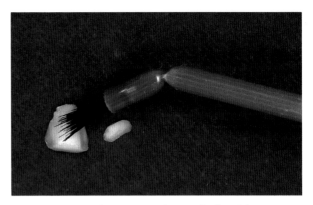

Fig 7–14 Bonding agent is applied, with a green brush, to the etched, silanated internal surface of the restoration.

Inlay/Onlay Placement Procedure

The porcelain restoration bonds to the tooth in a series of individual links:

- At the **tooth interface**, etched enamel micromechanically bonds with dental bonding agent.
- At the **restoration interface**, etched porcelain is made reactive via a silane, which mechanically and chemically bonds to an unfilled resin layer.
- These two **reactive interfaces** are joined by an optimized dual-cure hybrid composite resin luting agent.

Preparation of the Etched Porcelain Restoration for Luting

Cleaning the Restoration. The restoration is cleaned in the ultrasonic cleaner and then washed and dried. It is coated with a porcelain conditioner, which may be a standard enamel, 37% orthophosphoric acid etchant, or citric acid, for 1 minute. This is washed off with water for 20 seconds and dried with a chip syringe. The dried restoration is decontaminated by brushing on a ketone liquid (eg, Cavilax, ESPE-Premier; Dry-Bond, Den-Mat Corp) with a sable-hair brush. This process removes any contamination that might have occurred during the initial drying process with the chip syringe. The ketone liquid agent is allowed to vaporize, thus leaving a clean, dry, etched surface.

Silanation. The restoration is coated with a silane coupling agent, which makes the etched but nonreactive ceramic chemically bond to the composite resin luting agent. The silane is brushed on with a small, color-coordinated brush (eg, from Centrix, Inc) to cover the etched porcelain surfaces (Fig 7–13). The volatile silane is allowed to vaporize, thus leaving a thin layer of reactive silane on the surface. If it is not dry after 2 minutes, a stream of air can be directed approximately 4 to 6 inches above the restoration, parallel to its surface. This air flow is just passed across the surface and will speed up evaporation of the silane.

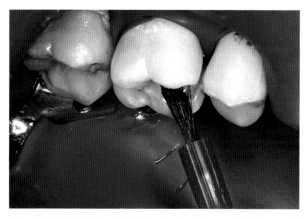

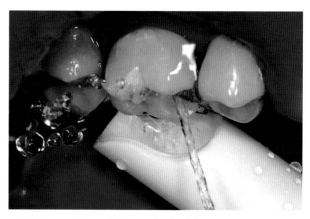

Fig 7–15 The tooth is treated with an etching acid placed on the enamel (with a red brush, Centrix, Inc) for 12 to 15 seconds. If a unietch system for enamel and dentin is used, 10% acid concentrate is applied for 30 seconds.

Fig 7–16 The acid is washed with water for approximately 20 seconds to ensure that all remnants are removed.

Application of Bonding Agent. A layer of unfilled resin or enamel bonding agent is applied with a disposable brush (Fig 7–14). This layer is then dispersed evenly, with the air syringe, over the etched, silanated surface of the restoration. This process can be combined into a single procedure because some manufacturers have combined the silane coupling agent and the resin bonding agent into a single liquid (eg, Ceriprime, Advanced Porcelain Restoration Kit, Den-Mat Corp). It is important to disperse this unfilled resin into an air-inhibited thin layer and to prevent pooling. Pooled resin that cures in the deeper layers can form tiny nodules that may prevent seating of the restoration. This etched, primed porcelain restoration is now ready for placement and should be kept in a container where it will not be contaminated or exposed to light (eg, Advanced Porcelain Restoration Kit, Den-Mat Corp; Resin Keeper, Cosmedent; Compo-Box, ESPE-Premier).

Preparation of the Tooth

Rubber Dam Isolation. It is essential to place the involved teeth under a rubber dam as this prevents moisture contamination and facilitates easy access for placement and finishing of the etched porcelain restoration. The rubber dam should encompass at least one tooth on either side of the prepared teeth. It should be of the extra-heavy variety, which helps to prevent seepage and displaces the interproximal soft tissues.

Cleaning the Cavity Preparation. If any try-in paste was used, the cavity preparation must be cleaned again with a wet slurry of flour pumice on a soft bristle brush (see Fig 7–8). This mixture is washed out and the preparation is dried with a chip syringe.

Etching. The tooth is treated with a liquid etchant (37% orthophosphoric acid) (Fig 7–15); a color-coordinated brush is used to eliminate confusion. The etching acid is placed on the surrounding enamel first, then the dentin, but *not over any glass-ionomer base.* The whole etching process should take between 12 and 15 seconds on enamel and less than 6 seconds on dentin. The action of the acid is stopped by using the chip syringe to wash out the acid (Fig 7–16). The newer unietch 10% orthophosphoric acids allow the acid to be used for 30 seconds over both enamel and dentin. The washing process should then take about 20 seconds to ensure that all remnants of the acid are removed. Gel acids usually require a longer period of washing.

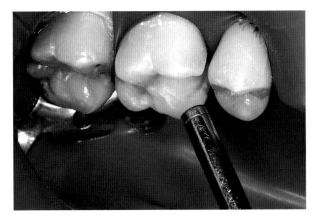

Fig 7–17 The preparation is blown dry of excess water with a chip syringe. The enamel should now appear frosted.

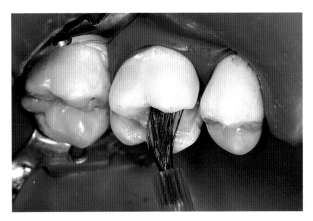

Fig 7–18 The dried area is decontaminated with a ketone liquid agent (used on a blue disposable brush).

Fig 7–19 The drying process is completed with an independent electric warm air source.

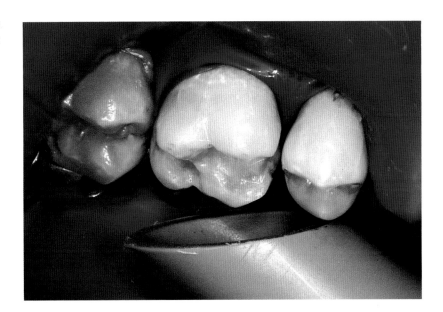

Drying. Drying is *traditionally* a three-phase procedure:

1. The washed preparation is dried with the dental unit's chip syringe (Fig 7–17). The etched enamel will appear to be frosted and white.
2. This frosted etched surface is decontaminated with a ketone liquid agent (Fig 7–18) (eg, Dry-Bond, Advanced Porcelain Restoration Kit, Den-Mat Corp; Cavilay, ESPE-Premier).
3. The decontaminated cavity preparation is dried with an independent source of warm air (Fig 7–19). Electric warm air dried at about 117°F to 120°F is preferable to warmed air from the dental unit, which uses the same contaminated air source.

Application of Dentin Bonding Agent

When a dentin bonding agent is used it should be mixed and brushed into the preparation and allowed to dry; at least five layers should be placed, especially when any dentin is exposed (Fig 7–20). Immediately following drying, a thin layer of the resin bonding agent should be painted over the entire surface area of the preparation (Fig 7–21). This should be gently dispersed into a thin film so that it does not pool and cure in certain areas and prevent seating of the restoration. The tooth surface is now reactive for the placement of the restoration.

Mixing and Placing the Composite Resin Luting Agent

It is important to use a dual-cure luting agent, which by its very nature necessitates mixing together either two pastes or a powder and a liquid (Fig 7–22). Neither system is ideal, because the mixing invariably incorporates air bubbles into the luting agent. This problem has been overcome in a system (eg, P.V.S., Jelenko) in which the catalyst for the curing process is incorporated into the resin bonding agent and activates the composite resin luting agent wherever the catalyst contacts the luting agent.

Separation

The tooth involved is isolated by placing ultrathin separating strips (eg, Advanced Porcelain Restoration Kit, Den-Mat Corp; Artus Corporation) in the interproximal spaces prior to placing the luting agent (Fig 7–23). It is essential to use these ultrafine strips to maintain separation to an absolute minimum. Celluloid strips or the dead-soft metal matrix bands are thicker and not as effective.

Application of the Composite Resin Luting Agent

The thin end of a strip of Super Floss (Oral B) is placed interproximally and apical to the finish line. The mixed composite resin luting agent is loaded into a syringe and injected into the cavity preparation (Fig 7–23). The etched fitting surface of the restoration is also coated with a thin layer of composite resin.

Seating the Restoration

The restoration is now gently manipulated into position and held firmly in place; composite resin should extrude around all margins. The use of ultrasonic vibrations (Siemens Sono-Cem) or any ultrasonic or piezoelectric scaler will greatly facilitate complete seating of the restoration by increasing the flow of even the most viscous of composite resin luting agents. A plastic end to the scaler tip is available, as metal tips tend to discolor the ceramic; a small piece of rubber dam also can act as an interface. The Super Floss beneath the contact point is drawn through to remove the excess resin interproximally. The inlay is pushed down firmly once again, which will extrude a further small bead of composite resin. The restoration is tacked in place by curing its center for about 30 seconds with a 14-mm tip placed in the curing light (Fig 7–24) (eg, Max-Light, LD Caulk; Demetron Curing Light, Demetron Research Corp). The inlay is held firmly in place, and the composite resin is then cured on each lateral surface for about 10 seconds. This will facilitate curing of the superficial layer of composite resin yet leave the underlying layer of resin still slightly doughy.

The gross excess composite resin is removed with a composite resin–trimming instrument (CRNT 12, NovaTech Series, Hu-Friedy). It is essential to ensure that a small bead of excess composite resin remains at the restoration–tooth surface interface. This bead ensures that, during further polymerization of the luting agent, and thus ongoing polymerization shrinkage of the luting agent, a void will not be created at the critical tooth-restoration interface.

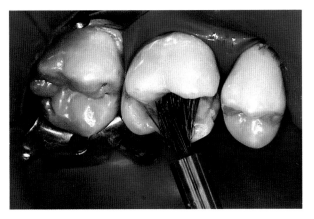

Fig 7–20 At least five layers of dentin bonding agent are placed over the entire cavity preparation and allowed to dry.

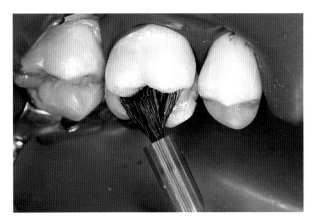

Fig 7–21 A thin layer of resin bonding agent is painted over the entire surface area of the preparation with a green disposable brush (Benda Brush, Centrix, Inc).

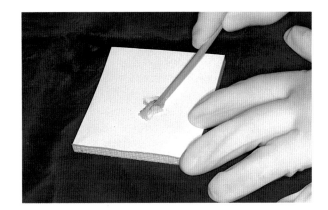

Fig 7–22 A dual-cure luting agent, which is either a paste-to-paste system or a powder-to-liquid system, is mixed.

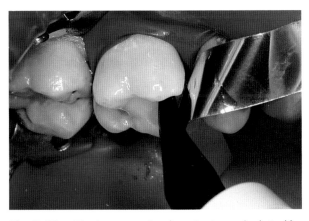

Fig 7–23 The interproximal contacts are isolated by separation with an ultrathin strip. The mixed composite resin luting agent is loaded into a composite resin syringe and injected into the internal aspects of the cavity preparation. Super Floss (Oral B) is placed interproximally and apical to the base of the box.

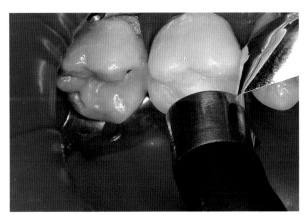

Fig 7–24 The inlay is cured in place for approximately 15 seconds on all aspects.

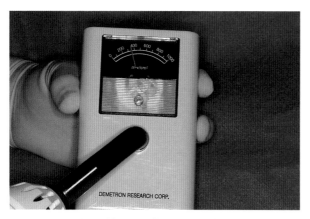

Fig 7–25 The efficacy of curing lights is evaluated on a metering unit (Demetron Research Corp).

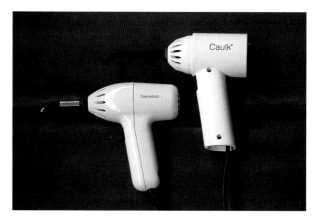

Fig 7–26 Two excellent light-curing sources with large-diameter curing tips that are sterilizable (Demetron Research Corp; LD Caulk).

Curing

The dual-cure composite resin is activated by white light and undergoes chemical polymerization.

Posterior restorations require the dual-cure system to ensure complete polymerization of all composite resin within the deeper aspects of the restoration.

The light-curing aspect of the dual-cure system is predicated on the following:

- **Time.** The longer the resin is exposed to the curing light (at least 2 minutes per surface), the greater the percentage of cure.
- **Shade of the resin.** Darker, more opaque resins tend to require greater lengths of time for the curing process to be completed.
- **Angle of contact.** If possible, the curing light should be directed at right angles to the resin interface. Placing the light at an oblique angle decreases its curing efficiency. Whenever optimal placement is not possible, the time exposure should be increased.
- **Distance.** To be most effective, the light source should be less than 1 mm from the surface of the composite resin. Sometimes this is not possible because of the depth of the preparation or the thickness of the restoration. The curing time must then be increased to compensate for the increased distance.

- **Luting agent composition.** Although the formulation of composite resin luting agents varies from manufacturer to manufacturer, the specific degree of cure for a given period of light exposure will vary among microfills, hybrids, and macrofills. In general, microfills allow less light to penetrate to the deeper layers.
- **Light-curing unit.** The light-curing unit (Fig 7–25) should be checked routinely every month to ensure that it is providing the required amount of photo energy to polymerize the resins. This is even more critical in those units with a fiberoptic wand where constant manipulation of the wand breaks some of the bundle fibers, thus decreasing the efficacy of its curing power. Even the self-contained units must be checked to ensure that the output of the bulb is adequate. A calibrating device for checking the efficacy of light-curing units is available (Cure Rite, Efos). Or the efficacy can simply be tested by placing a dark microfill composite resin in a 2-mm-thick ring or washer and curing from the top. The composite resin on the undersurface should be checked for hardness by scraping with a curet or scaler.

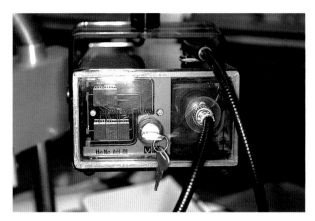

Fig 7–27 The argon soft laser (Framatome Prototype) has been used experimentally to expedite the curing process.

In posterior restorations it is useful to use two curing lights simultaneously. This allows energy from both buccal and lingual surfaces to penetrate simultaneously to the deeper aspects of the resin, thereby decreasing the chances that unpolymerized luting agent will be left in those areas.

Many lights come with a variety of different curing tips, but a 12- to 15-mm tip is most useful because the light should not be moved during the curing process in an attempt to cover all surfaces simultaneously. The tip must be kept in one position for the entire curing period before it is moved to another area. The larger tip therefore works more effectively, provided that the access opening to the light source in the gun is as wide as the tip (Fig 7–26).

Laser Curing

An argon soft laser (Fig 7–27) has been used experimentally and appears to be very effective for curing composite resin. The depth of penetration is considerably greater, and the degree of cure is more rapid and complete. The laser may also facilitate use of a purely light-polymerized luting agent, thereby avoiding mixing and decreasing time.

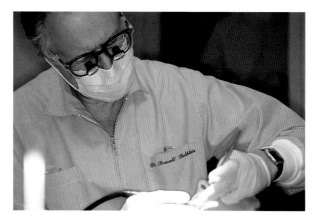

Fig 7–28a Use of magnification is as essential during the finishing procedures as it is during the cavity preparation.

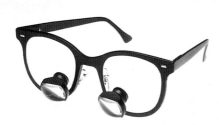

Fig 7–28b Wide-angled rectangular × 2.5 magnifying glasses (Designs For Vision, Inc).

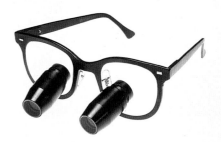

Fig 7–28c Magnifying glasses with a narrower field of vision but with × 4.5 magnification (Designs For Vision, Inc).

Finishing

All finishing procedures are greatly enhanced by the use of some form of magnification (Fig 7–28a). The magnification device can be as simple as the flip-down type of × 2 magnification clip-on lenses, or it can be the more efficacious × 2.5 wide-field magnifying telescopes with a focal lens that is adjustable for specific working needs and different interpupillary distances (Fig 7–28b).

Depending on the magnification needs, the strength can be increased, but the field of vision is slightly decreased (Fig 7–28c). Following complete polymerization of at least 2 minutes on each surface of the restoration or tooth, any remaining composite resin can be peeled away with the flattened interproximal aspect or with the sickle end of the composite resin–trimming instrument (eg, CRNT 12, NovaTech Series, Hu-Friedy).

The finishing procedures are best accomplished with a series of microfine diamond strips and multibladed carbides specifically designed for the finishing process. A 30-blade finishing carbide (Brasseler Corp) is run along the porcelain-tooth interface to remove the tiny bead of composite resin remaining on the occlusal surface. Alternatively, a yellow-band 15-μm finishing diamond (E.T. Series, Brasseler Corp) can be used (Fig 7–29). If the inlay has not seated completely and there is some porcelain flash beyond the margin of the cavity, this may need to be machined down to the level of the tooth with an E.T. finishing diamond. All instruments are used with a copious water spray so as not to overheat the luting resin and/or dental pulp. In general, the carbide is used first, as it will remove the softer resin without affecting the adjacent porcelain or tooth.

The interproximal areas are cleared of excess resin with a 30-blade finishing carbide (4-mm E.T. or microfine diamond, Brasseler) (Fig 7–30) used buccolingually as well as occlusoapically to trim all exposed marginal areas. The interproximal areas are then checked with an explorer as well as with a length of unwaxed floss to ensure that there is smooth transition between the remaining tooth surface and the restoration. If the profile of the enamel does not appear to be confluent with that of the porcelain, the porcelain may need adjusting and reshaping with a microfine finishing diamond. The reciprocating handpiece, which has varying sizes and grits of diamond tips, is an excellent device for clearing interproximal excess (Fig 7–31).

Occlusal Adjustment

Once the inlay has been bonded into position and cured completely, the occlusal relationships can be evaluated (Fig 7–32). This process is not possible until all the excess composite resin has been removed from the surface of the restoration. Generally it is desirable to see a series of markings down the central fossae of the teeth in both the maxillary and mandibular posterior segments. However, if the markings occur only on the teeth where the restorations were placed, then it is necessary to make an appropriate occlusal adjustment. The adjustment can be made either to the restoration just placed or to the opposing arch. This necessitates clinical judgment by the clinician, who must take into account the harmony and continuity of form of the line angles of the supporting cusps and the central fossae of all the teeth in the segments being restored. If it is decided the porcelain should be adjusted, this should be done with either a DOS-1 or DOS-1-EF microfine diamond (Brasseler). The porcelain should then be polished with an impregnated polishing wheel (Porcelain Laminate Polishing Kit, Shofu) (Fig 7–33).

After the occlusion is confirmed, the restoration is adjusted, first for maximum intercuspation or centric occlusion and then for lateral excursive movements of the mandible.

The restorations should not develop contacts and markings on the inner aspects of the cusps during lateral or protrusive movements of the mandible (Fig 7–32).

Porcelain has the potential to wear a natural opposing occlusion at a far greater rate than either natural tooth substance or gold. Although this wear can take place to a minor extent during functional activities, it predominates during parafunctional habits. Therefore, the early contacts beyond the centric occlusion markings in any direction should be eliminated. This requires changing the functional outer aspects of the opposing cusps or hollowing out the central fossa of the restoration. When the occlusal adjustment is being performed, it is useful to develop the centric holding stops in one color and the lateral excursive movements in a different color. This makes it easy to maintain the centric holds while the differently colored markings associated with lateral movements are adjusted.

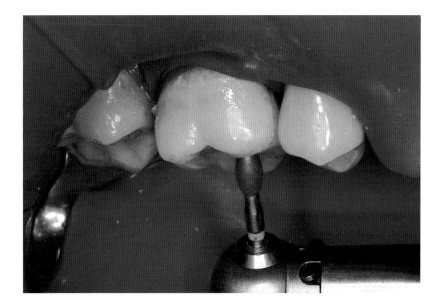

Fig 7–29 A 30-blade finishing carbide (E.T. Series, no. 6, Brasseler Corp) or microfine diamond is used to remove excess composite resin occlusally and to finish the margin.

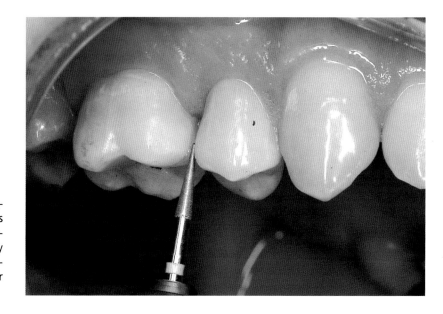

Fig 7–30 A microfine 3-mm diamond (E.T. Series, no. 3 yellow) is used to remove excess resin interproximally. A 30-fluted similarly shaped carbide can be used to finish the margin (E.T. 6-U.F., Brasseler Corp).

Fig 7–31 Interproximal excess of composite resin, particularly at the base of the box, can be removed and the area can be polished with a reciprocating handpiece and diamond tips (Profin, Weissman Technology International).

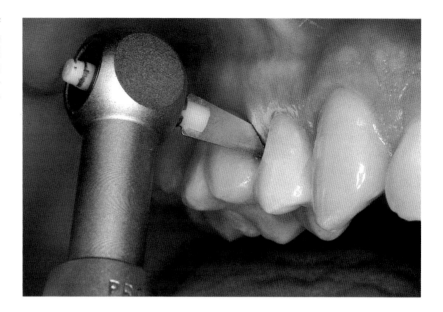

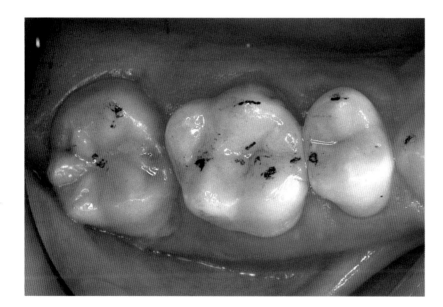

Fig 7–32 The occlusal scheme is verified by using black for centric occlusion and red for lateral excursive movements of the mandible. In general, there should be no red markings on the inner aspects of the cusps on either side of the central fossa of the porcelain restoration.

Polishing

The restoration in its entirety now needs polishing. Any areas that have been occlusally adjusted as well as all marginal aspects must be polished. The easiest way to do this is with ceramic-polishing points (Fig 7–33) followed by a rubber cup with diamond-impregnated paste (Fig 7–34). It is important to polish not only the occlusal surface, which is clearly evident, but also the interproximal areas, to prevent them from becoming depositories for microbial plaque. In the interproximal areas it is useful to use the reciprocating action of the Profin diamond-impregnated flexible files. The interproximal areas are finally polished with a composite resin–polishing strip (eg, 3M; Cosmedent) and are checked to see that floss does not catch in any direction (Fig 7–35), especially apico-occlusally. If the interproximal areas do not permit the passage of floss, they can be cleared with one of the metal diamond-impregnated strips prior to the polishing procedure (Fig 7–36).

The original failing amalgam restoration (Fig 7–37a) and its replacement, a porcelain inlay (Fig 7–37b), can be compared.

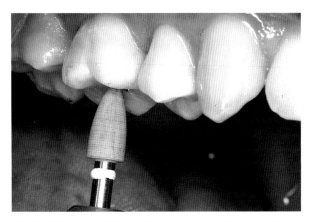

Fig 7–33 Porcelain-polishing points (Porcelain Laminate Polishing Kit, Shofu) are used to finish the marginal aspect of the restoration and any occlusally adjusted areas.

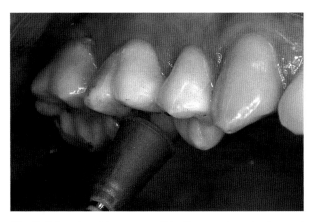

Fig 7–34 A rubber cup with diamond paste is used to develop the final luster and polish of the etched porcelain restoration.

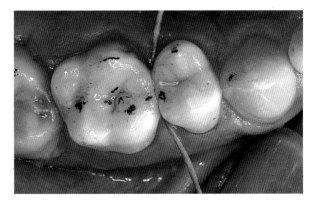

Fig 7–35 Interproximal areas are checked to ensure that the contact points are open and that floss does not catch when passed through the contact areas.

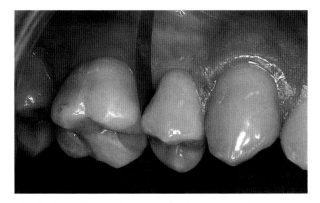

Fig 7–36 If floss does catch, the area of the tooth is stripped, first with a diamond finishing strip (eg, Compo-Strip, Premier Dental Products; G-C Finishing Strips, G-C International) and then with a composite resin–finishing strip.

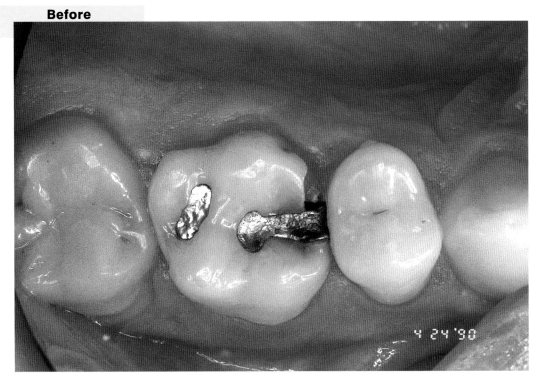

Fig 7–37a Preoperative occlusal view of failing amalgam restoration.

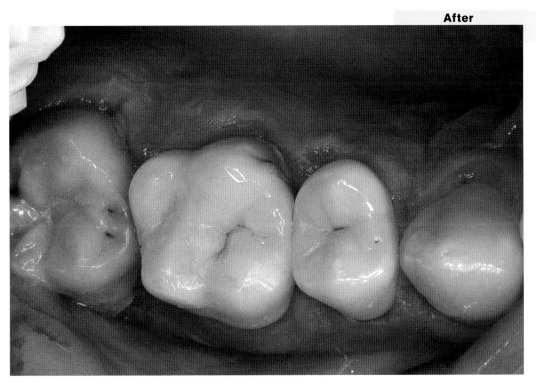

Fig 7–37b Postoperative view of replacement porcelain inlay. Occlusal view of the two polished inlays: the occlusal inlay in the distal fossa and the occlusal compound restoration.

Cast-Ceramic Systems and Other Alternatives

8

Conventional porcelain is extremely brittle and has great potential to fracture during function because microscopic defects (inherent in the ceramic) can occur under loading. Bonding the ceramic to a metal substructure alleviates this problem but tends to compromise esthetics. An alternative solution when using an all-ceramic restoration is to incorporate various fiber-reinforcing systems to decrease the fracture potential. The controlled microcrystallization of a dual-phase glass-ceramic system produces a significant increase in the fracture resistance of the ceramic material, making glass ceramics an attractive alternative.

Cast Ceramics (Dicor)

Over the years castable glass-ceramic systems have proved to be a viable alternative ceramic system. The first of these castable glass-ceramic systems was introduced by Dentsply International-

al and developed by Dow Corning. The systems have been used for a variety of different clinical situations, including crowns, porcelain laminate veneers, all-ceramic fixed partial dentures, cores for ceramic crowns, as well as inlays and onlays. The immediate advantage of this type of ceramic process over the conventional porcelain systems is that it utilizes the conventional waxing on a die and casting techniques similar to the conventional lost-wax technique used for cast-metal restorations.

Following tooth preparation and impression making of the compromised tooth (Fig 8–1), an accurately indexed working cast with individual dies is developed. Wax is then formed to reproduce the desired tooth anatomy, incorporating occlusal harmony and function with the opposing arch (Fig 8–2). The patterns are finished and accurately fitted in their entirety before being removed from the die, sprued, and invested (Fig 8–3). The phosphate-bonded type of investment is specific for the system used, but the process is similar. Stucco is first carefully painted onto the sprued pattern with a soft camel-hair brush; then the rest of the investment is flowed and

Fig 8–1 Preoperative view of a compromised amalgam restoration that needs replacement.

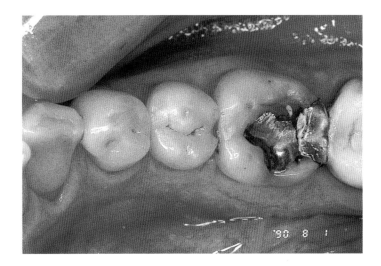

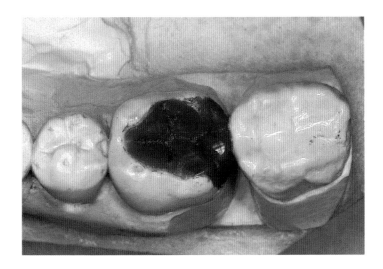

Fig 8–2 The restorations are waxed up in their entirety on the indexed working casts and dies.

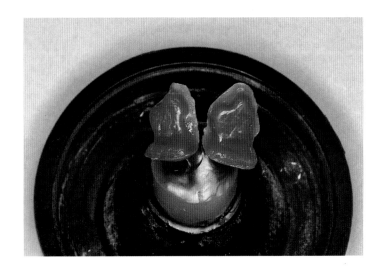

Fig 8–3 The patterns are finished entirely on the dies, removed, and then sprued for the investment procedure.

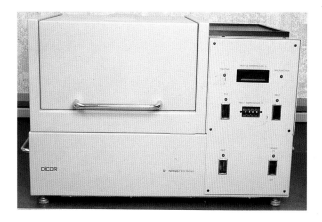

Fig 8–4 The casting ring is placed in the centrifugal casting instrument, which delivers the molten glass into the pattern.

vibrated into the respective casting ring carefully, to avoid entrapment of air bubbles.

Once the investment has set, the casting ring is placed in a burnout furnace, where it is gently heated to 350°C and held at this temperature for 30 to 45 minutes to volatilize the wax pattern. The temperature is then increased to 900°C to bring the crucible investment complex to the correct casting temperature.

When the casting ring has reached the correct temperature, a specific centrifugal casting instrument is used. The single-use crucible containing the casting glass pellet is heated within the electronic muffle of the casting arm until molten. In the Dicor System (Dentsply International), for instance, the temperature reached is approximately 1,365°C. At this time the casting ring is transferred to the modified centrifugal casting instrument (Fig 8–4), which delivers the molten glass into the pattern.

The amorphous glass castings are divested (Fig 8–5), cleaned of any extraneous materials, and checked for accuracy on the respective casts. If they appear to be correct, they are transferred to the ceramming oven (Fig 8–6), which changes the amorphous crystalline structure of the clear cast glass into the semicrystalline opaque ceramic (Fig 8–7). In this process, the glass is heated for 105 minutes to 1,075°C and held there for ap-

proximately 6 hours. It is then slowly cooled for an hour to between 400°C and 500°C, thus completing the ceramming process.

The cast-ceramic restorations are then finished, smoothed, and polished and are refitted to the individual dies. In the cast-glass system, it is advisable for the castings to be clinically tried in the patient's mouth at a separate appointment so that they can be adjusted intraorally for any occlusal discrepancies and to conform to the patient's stomatognathic system. Interproximal contact relations should also be adjusted to allow complete seating. Once this is completed to the clinician's satisfaction, the restorations are returned to the laboratory, where they can be surface stained and characterized (Fig 8–8) by using a specific Dicor ceramic-shading system. In the cast-glass laminate veneers, some degree of color modification is also derived from the light-activated, color-coordinated composite resin luting agent, but in the thicker cast-glass inlay, this feature is somewhat limited.

The internal fitting surfaces of the restorations are etched with 10% ammonium-bifluoride to improve their bonding strength to the composite resin and the tooth. The restorations are then ready for placement (Fig 8–9), in the same manner as described in chapter 7, with one of the composite resin luting systems.

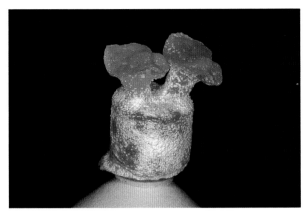

Fig 8–5 The amorphous glass castings are removed from the investment before the sprues are cut off.

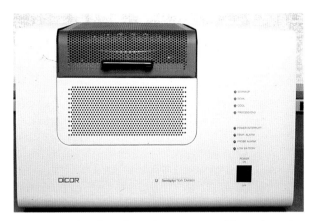

Fig 8–6 The fitted castings are transferred to the ceramming oven to undergo the transformation process from crystallization to opaque ceramic.

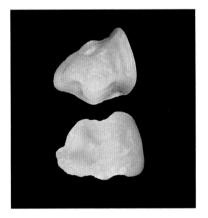

Fig 8–7 Cerammed opaque castings prior to finishing and retrofitting.

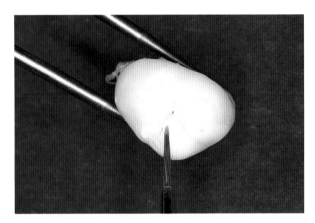

Fig 8–8 The fitted restorations are surface stained and characterized with the ceramic-shading system.

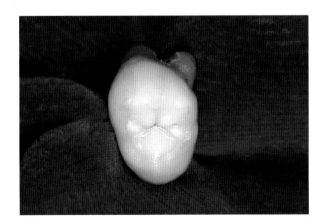

Fig 8–9 Completed restorations prior to cementation.

Advantages

- The fit of cast-glass restorations reportedly supersedes that of conventional porcelain. This decreases the amount of resin luting agent at the margins, in turn decreasing the potential for ditching.
- The wear on the opposing occlusion is predicted to be less than that of conventional porcelains.
- The thermal cycling properties of cast glass approximate those of enamel.
- Flexural strength is reportedly greater than it is for conventional porcelain.

Disadvantages

- The colorant is a surface stain, hence any grinding on the restoration leaves an unesthetic opaque white area.
- An additional chairside visit is necessary to fit and adjust the contacts, anatomic form, and occlusion prior to staining. Once stained, the surface cannot be adjusted without compromising the esthetics.
- The whole process is technique-sensitive, from the casting of the inlays through the staining of the cerammed restorations.

Pressed-Ceramic Systems (IPS Empress)

A newer material of the all-ceramic type, which is not cast but injection molded, is IPS Empress (Ivoclar-Vivadent). This system uses high-temperature pressing of a preceramed glass ceramic with hydrostatic pressure in a vacuum unit. The inlay or onlay is modeled in wax on a conventional die system (Fig 8–10). The wax pattern is then sprued and invested (Fig 8–11) in a special material to allow for the injection molding of the glass ceramic. The ring is placed in a cold burnout oven and progressively heated to 850°C and held at this temperature for 90 minutes for wax burnout and heat saturation. The ring is then ready for placement in the pressing furnace (Fig 8–12), which is in a standby mode at a temperature of 700°C. One or two preceramed pellets of the desired color (Fig 8–13) are placed in the center of the sprue former.

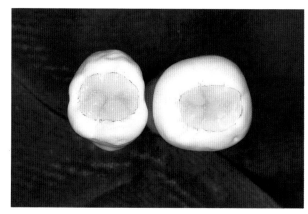

Fig 8–10 In IPS Empress ceramic systems, the restoration is molded in tooth-colored wax on a conventional die system.

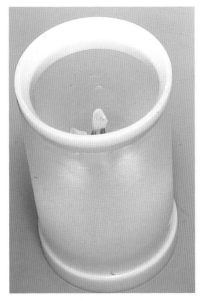

Fig 8–11 The wax pattern is sprued and invested.

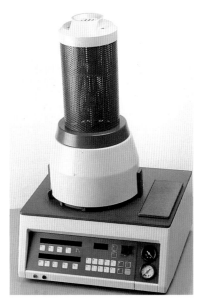

Fig 8–12 The ring is placed in the IPS Empress hydrostatically-controlled furnace (Ivoclar-Vivadent).

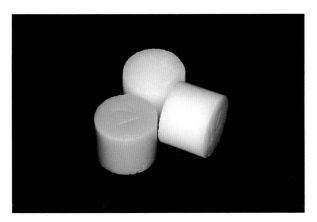

Fig 8–13 Ceramic pellets in the specifically selected base shade.

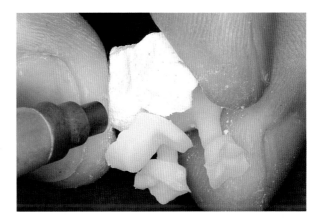

Fig 8–14 The pressed-ceramic restorations are removed from the investment and cleaned.

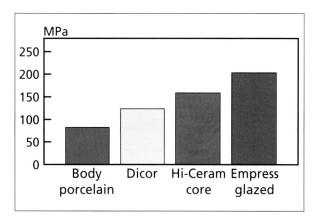

Fig 8–15 Three-point flexural strength of IPS Empress pressed ceramic compared to other glass-ceramic materials (Dicor, Dentsply International; Hi-Ceram, Vident) and traditional body porcelain. (Internal data from Ivoclar North America, Inc; measurements performed in accordance with ISO 6872 for dental ceramics.)

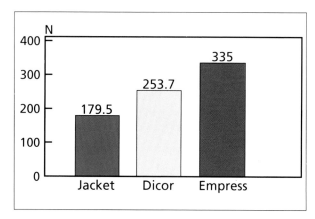

Fig 8–16 Results of a study (Ludwig 1991) comparing fracture resistance of IPS Empress, Dicor, and traditional jacket crowns. Multiple crowns were fabricated and subjected to a 30-degree axial load until fracture occurred. (Adapted from Ludwig 1991.)

Once the process is initiated, the temperature in the furnace elevates to 1,100°C under a vacuum. A pneumatic plunger on the automated program of the Empress oven begins to inject the molten ceramic into the form of the restoration left by the wax burnout. Once these voids are completely filled, the plunger maintains the hydrostatic pressure during the entire cooling cycle. The vacuum and heating are turned off automatically, and the chamber containing the mold is opened so the mold can be removed. The mold is allowed to bench cool to room temperature before being removed from the investment and cleaned off with a glass bead air abrader (Fig 8-14). The sprue is cut off with a diamond rotary disk. The pressed-ceramic restoration is tried on the die and adjusted for contact relations and occlusion before being finished with microfine rotary diamonds.

Composition

IPS Empress pressed ceramic is manufactured from two basic glasses, which during processing are transformed from an amorphous glass into a heterogenous glass ceramic with smaller, more densely dispersed microcrystals. Because of the difference in coefficients of thermal expansion of the glass matrix and the microcrystals, the overall ceramic is maintained in a state of compression, which results in a significant increase in strength (Figs 8–15 and 8–16).

The ingots are preshaped and available in the full Vita and Ivoclar color range to more closely approximate the base shade of the desired restoration. They are also available in varying degrees of opacity.

Staining

The pressed-ceramic material is somewhat translucent, so that the color of the underlying tooth structure can be transmitted through it. Therefore, the die material is available in seven different dentinal shades (Fig 8–13). The shade of the prepared tooth (ie, the dentin) is determined with a specially formulated shade guide, the chromoscope (Fig 8–17), following tooth preparation. The restoration can then be completed in one of two ways.

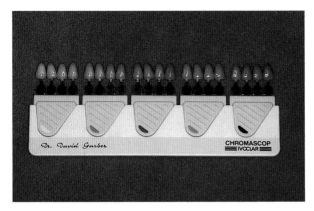

Fig 8–17 Specially formulated shade guide.

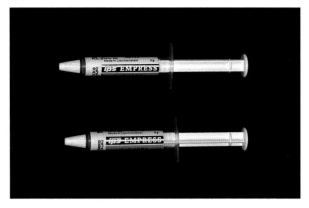

Fig 8–18 Specifically formulated shading porcelains already prepared in syringes.

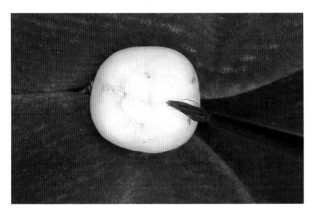

Fig 8–19 The restoration is painted and characterized.

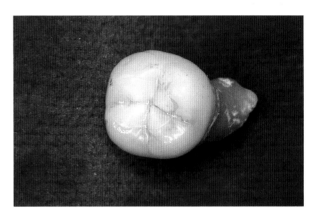

Fig 8–20 Intricately characterized IPS Empress restoration.

Surface Staining Technique. This is used most often in the posterior region for inlays, onlays, and some posterior crowns. The pressed-ceramic ideally waxed restoration is adjusted for contacts and is characterized with a specifically developed shading porcelain (Fig 8–18). This is painted onto the base-colored restoration (Fig 8–19). The firing cycle is only 2 minutes at 850°C using vacuum. The shaded restoration is tried on the dentin-shaded die; glycerine is used to transmit the color of the die through to the final restoration. The shading may require between two and four firings for the final intrinsic characterization to be developed (Fig 8–20).

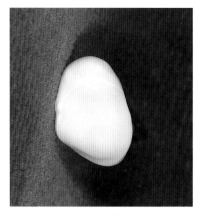

Fig 8–21 Incompletely waxed IPS Empress core before the final characterization is layered in.

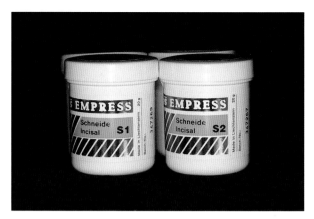

Fig 8–22 IPS Empress porcelains for layering.

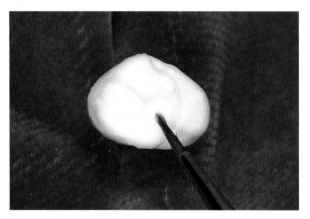

Fig 8–23 The incisal enamel porcelains are layered onto the basic core of pressed ceramic.

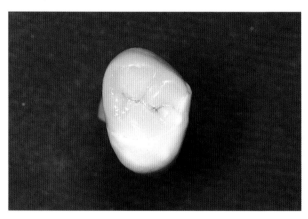

Fig 8–24 The completed restoration comprises a core of pressed ceramic and layered porcelains.

Layering Technique. An alternative technique to optimize esthetics for crowns or inlays may require layering over an I.P.S. Empress anatomic coping (Fig 8–21), a concept developed by Willi Geller. The restoration is not waxed to full contour, so that a sufficient space can be left after ceramic pressing for the layering on of incisal translucency and individual characterizations. If insufficient space exists, a cutback of the ceramic core is possible. A specifically developed porcelain with a lower coefficient of thermal expansion is used for the layering (Fig 8–22). Thus the porcelain layered over the basic pressed porcelain is maintained in a state of compression, which adds strength to the system. The incisal and enamel layers (Fig 8–23) are baked separately on the core before final stain characterization and finishing (Fig 8–24).

Advantages of Pressed-Ceramic Systems

- The pressed-ceramic system involves relatively simple processing procedures that accurately reproduce the waxed pattern. The cerammed restorations have a high degree of stability during subsequent shading or layering techniques.
- The precerammed porcelain has a high degree of flexural tensile strength (exceeding 200 MPa). This makes the material adequate for most normal restorations, let alone those bonded to the underlying tooth structure.

- The versatility of the process allows for the development of very esthetic restorations ranging from inlays and onlays to full crowns and laminate veneers, even in very thin sections of only 1 mm (Figs 8–25a to d).
- The lost-wax technique and ceramic injection molding allow for accurate fit.
- The preshaded base ingots with two different characterization techniques allow achievement of excellent harmony and blending with adjacent teeth.

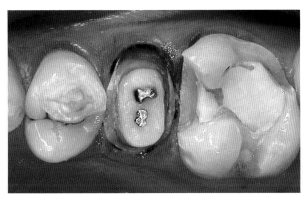

Fig 8–25a Three teeth prepared to receive *(left to right)* a tiny buccal cusp tip on the first premolar, an all-ceramic crown on the second premolar, and a mesio-occlusolingual inlay on the molar.

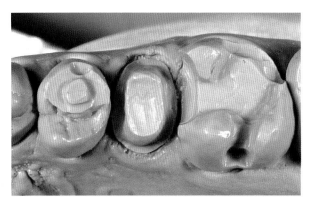

Fig 8–25b Master cast showing the preparations for the tiny onlay, the full-crown, and the inlay.

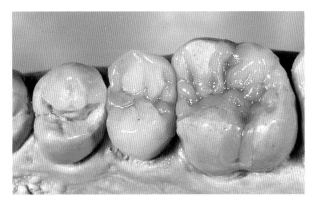

Fig 8–25c Anatomic shaded waxup of three restorations on the master cast.

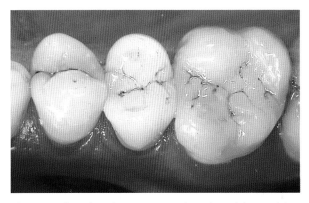

Fig 8–25d The three restorations luted in position show the versatility of the pressed-ceramic system for different types of restorations and excellent potential for matching tooth structure. (Photographs courtesy of Arnold Wohlwend.)

Reinforced Conventional Porcelain

When large amounts of tooth substance have been lost (Fig 8–26), fabrication of a conventional porcelain restoration becomes somewhat complex. The variation in porcelain thicknesses on the different tooth surfaces results in differences in sintering shrinkage deformation and poor marginal adaptation. Conventionally, an even layer of porcelain is created by building up the cavity preparation with a glass-ionomer or similar base. This modification of the cavity preparation should result in even dimensions of all surfaces and hence even thicknesses of ceramic on all surfaces. Unfortunately, some of the base materials, such as glass-ionomer cement, are inherently too weak for extremely large buildups.

An alternative method of solving this problem was developed so that the ideal cavity form does not have to be redeveloped with glass-ionomer buildups and teeth still do not have to be restored with full-coverage restorations. An impression of the uneven cavity preparation is made and a cast with dies is poured to prevent distortion. A base of one of the reinforced aluminous ceramic cores is first built up in this large cavity preparation, which will support the surface layers of porcelain in the subsequent firings and prevent warpage (Fig 8–27).

One such system that is reportedly somewhat stronger and more stable than conventional porcelain is Hi-Ceram (Vident). A stronger glass-refilled ceramic system (In-Ceram, Vident) will also effectively support large amounts of porcelain. These core materials are built up as the base to the conventional ceramic (Fig 8–27) and are inherently stable so that, with subsequent firings, the disproportionate thicknesses of the porcelain and the repeated firing processes do not result in distortion of the overlying ceramic (Fig 8–28).

This stable base concept can also be used with an underlying cast substructure of metal ceramic that is waxed, cast, and shaped (Fig 8–29), leaving sufficient thickness for an opaquing medium and the ceramic (Fig 8–30). Depending on the type of metal used, this restoration can be etched and then bonded to the dentin and remaining tooth structure as described in Chapter 7.

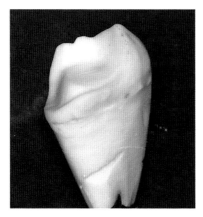

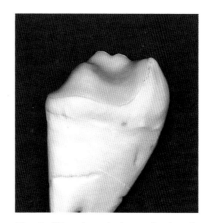

Fig 8–26 Preparation showing no potential for an even thickness of porcelain, because of variation in the amounts of lost tooth structure.

Fig 8–27 A reinforced aluminous ceramic core placed in the base of an excessively large cavity preparation stabilizes subsequent layers of porcelain during repetitive firing cycles.

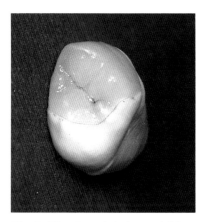

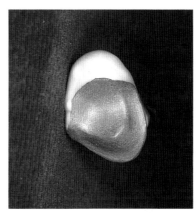

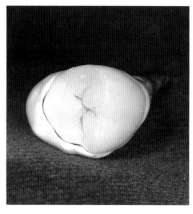

Fig 8–28 Porcelain is overlaid on the reinforced ceramic core to complete the natural form of the tooth.

Fig 8–29 Metal substructure on internal fitting aspects of the cavity preparation prior to placement of porcelain.

Fig 8–30 The completed hybrid restoration with metal reinforcing the overlying ceramic.

Composite Resin Inlays— An Alternative to Ceramic Inlays

9

Howard Strassler/Leonard Litkowski

In recent years several manufacturers have introduced indirectly fabricated and combined direct-indirect composite resin inlay systems. There are many reasons for using these new composite resin inlay systems, including their good adaptation at the cavosurface margins, especially the gingival margin; their reduced polymerization shrinkage compared to direct composite resin placement; easy manipulation of material out of the mouth; and excellent characterization and adjustment of the occlusal surface.

These new systems use a dual-cure technique of light polymerization combined with a continued heat hardening and curing in special ovens. Some manufacturers offer a light-curing oven for the fabrication of composite resin inlays. Once the inlay is cured it is then bonded to the tooth structure with a light and chemical cure bonding system. These systems and the type of curing recommended are listed in Table 9–1.

Treatment Planning

The decision to use composite resin inlays for the esthetic restoration of posterior teeth is based in part on a thorough evaluation of the existing intraoral conditions, the status of the tooth to be restored, and time and cost considerations. In many instances the composite resin inlay can be used interchangeably with directly placed composite resin restorations. The indications for composite resin posterior inlays include:

- Restoration of conservative cavity preparations that have an isthmus of less than one third the cuspal distance
- Replacement of posterior composite resin restorations that have been successful for a long period of time but now need routine replacement because of fracture, wear, or recurrent caries
- Replacement of existing metallic restorations for esthetic reasons that do not require the complete onlaying of the occlusal surface

Table 9–1 *Composite Resin Inlay Systems*

Name of System	Type of System	Type of Curing	Manufacturer
Brillant DI	Direct-indirect	Light/heat	Coltene-Whaledent
Clearfil CR Inlay	Indirect	Light/heat	Kuraray
Concept	Indirect	Light/heat	Vivadent
Conquest	Indirect	Light	Jeneric/Pentron
Dentacolor	Indirect	Light	Kulzer
EOS	Indirect	Light	Vivadent
True Vitality	Direct-indirect or indirect	Light/heat	Den-Mat Corp
Visio-Gem	Indirect	Light/vacuum	ESPE-Premier

- Esthetic restoration of teeth in patients who have a diagnosis of bruxism or clenching and exhibit mild to moderate wear on the opposing dentition

Composite resin inlays can be used in maxillary and mandibular premolars and molars that fulfill these criteria.

Preparation Design

The preparation design for composite resin inlays is the same as described in chapter 4. Most importantly, the path of draw must be adequate for removal of the inlay in either the direct or indirect method and yet maintain an adequate bulk of material to prevent fracture of the resin. Important features in the preparation design are slight flaring of the proximal margins, a slight bevel (created with a gingival margin trimmer) on the gingival cavosurface margin, and no occlusal bevel. Cavosurface margins should not be placed in centric holding areas of the occlusion because of the susceptibility to fracture of these areas. The preparation is accomplished with a long, smooth tapered fissure bur or tapered diamonds (eg, E.T. Series, Brasseler Corp) so that the walls of the cavity preparation are relatively smooth and free of irregularities and undercuts.

The preparation is slightly overtapered compared to that of a cast-gold inlay and has a combined divergent angle of both buccal and lingual walls of 15 to 20 degrees.

Preparation pulpal depth should be at least 1.5 mm and will usually end about 0.5 mm into the dentin. However, it is mandatory that the thickness of the material be at least 1.0 mm in non–load-bearing areas and a minimum of 1.5 mm in areas with occlusal contact. Axial depth of the preparation will be determined by the extent of the proximal caries or the previous preparation with the defective restorative material being replaced. For preparations with less than 1.0 mm of dentin over the pulp, it is recommended that a light-curing glass-ionomer liner, such as LC Zionomer (Den-Mat Corp), Vitrebond (3M), or G-C Liner (G-C International), be used as a base. Shade selection should be made prior to tooth preparation to obtain a better match. Commonly, however, an existing metallic restoration is being replaced and it is therefore necessary to match the shade to an adjacent tooth. If a large number of restorations are to be performed in a given quadrant, the shade can be selected for the optimum color change, similar to the shade selection for anterior bonding. Because resin materials are translucent, the restoration will acquire some of the original shading of the tooth, and this can be used to advantage for a more natural appearance of the tooth-restoration interface.

Provisionalization

The preparation is provisionalized with self-curing acrylic resin. The rubber dam is removed for the fabrication of the provisional restoration. For an inlay, the provisional restoration can be constructed directly on the prepared tooth in the patient's mouth. A light coat of the patient's own saliva may be painted into the preparation to act as a lubricant. A stainless steel matrix band with the retainer and wooden wedge can be used to control the acrylic resin flow during placement.

Two drops of monomer liquid are placed into a dappen dish and enough powder is added to form a runny mix of acrylic resin. When the mix acquires slightly less flow, a disposable brush (eg, BendaBrush, Centrix, Inc) is used to paint some of the acrylic resin into the tooth preparation, covering the gingival wall. When the mix becomes doughy, it is placed into the cavity preparation with an angled flat plastic instrument. The patient should close into maximum intercuspation and go through all mandibular excursive movements to establish the parameters of an occlusal form. Once the acrylic resin starts to harden, the matrix retainer is loosened and the restoration is worked up and down within the preparation to prevent it from locking into the cavity when complete polymerization is reached.

After polymerization, the matrix and acrylic resin restoration are removed from the tooth. All the margins of the preparation in the acrylic resin restoration undersurface are evaluated. The excess acrylic resin is trimmed with acrylic resin burs and abrasive disks. A final polish is placed with a prophylaxis cup with pumice.

After the finishing stage, the restoration is placed back into the tooth preparation to evaluate the fit and marginal adaptation of the restoration. Articulating paper is used to check the occlusion and make any adjustments that are necessary to maintain the occlusion and proximal contacts. The restoration is cemented with a non–eugenol-based temporary cement such as Provicell (Septodont) or TempBond N.E. (Kerr/Sybron). A eugenol-containing temporary cement may have a negative effect on the adhesive procedures and materials used for bonding the composite resin inlay to place.

Fabrication of the Composite Resin Inlay

The fabrication technique for the composite resin inlay depends on the specific system of materials being used. Two different fabrication techniques are available: a combined *direct-indirect technique* and an *indirect technique.*

Direct-Indirect Technique

For this technique, the composite resin inlay is fabricated directly on the tooth preparation in the mouth and then the inlay is removed and cured in a curing oven. During the fabrication it is recommended that a rubber dam be used to isolate the area and to avoid salivary and hemorrhagic contamination of the composite resin restorative material. Two commercial systems can be used with this technique: the Brilliant Direct Inlay System (Coltene-Whaledent) and the True Vitality System (Den-Mat Corp).

Lubrication of the Inlay Preparation. Once the inlay preparation has been completed (Fig 9–1), the tooth and cavity preparation are liberally painted with a lubricant (eg, Separator, Coltene-Whaledent) on a disposable brush (Fig 9–2). This lubricant is compatible with the hybrid composite resin inlay restorative material and will allow inlay removal after intraoral light curing.

Matrix and Wedge Placement. A retainerless, contoured, clear matrix (eg, CureThru Matrix, ESPE-Premier) is placed and clear reflecting wedges (eg, Cure-Thru Wedge, ESPE-Premier) are placed at the interproximal gingival margins. The wedges are firmly placed to create rapid separation of the teeth, compensating for thickness of the Mylar matrix band and allowing for the interproximal contact between the inlay and adjacent teeth. The lubricant is lightly thinned with a gentle air stream from a tri-syringe.

Composite Resin Inlay Material Placement. The hybrid composite resin is placed into the inlay preparation by taking the high-viscosity resin paste, placing it into the proximal box, and

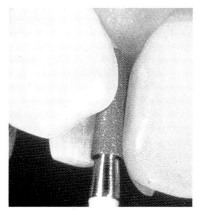 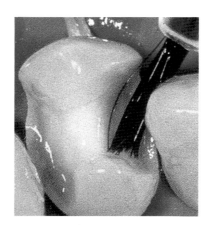 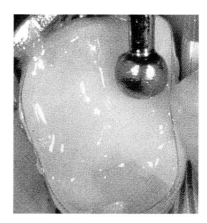

Fig 9–1 Composite resin inlay preparation created with tapered fissure diamond; note a divergence of walls of 15 to 20 degrees. (Figures 9–1 through 9–7 courtesy of Coltene-Whaledent.)

Fig 9–2 The cavity preparation is painted with a lubricant compatible with the composite resin inlay material; this facilitates removal of the inlay after light curing.

Fig 9–3 The preparation has been filled with the composite resin. The occlusal surface is shaped and the margins are adapted with a ball burnisher that has been slightly wetted with resin adhesive.

gently condensing it with a ball burnisher. After the composite resin has been placed in the proximal box, the occlusal portion of the preparation is completely filled and gently condensed with a ball burnisher that has been lightly coated with a resin adhesive to deter the composite resin from sticking to the end of the burnisher (Fig 9–3).

Once again, firm pressure is placed on the reflecting wedges to guarantee rapid separation of the teeth and to avoid creating gingival excess of the composite resin inlay material. The end of a curved light-curing tip is placed firmly on the end of the reflecting wedge and the interproximal area is cured for 60 seconds. The interproximal surfaces are cured from the facial and lingual aspects; then the occlusal surface is cured for 60 seconds also (Fig 9–4).

Inlay Removal. After the completion of light curing, the inlay must be removed from the preparation. A scaler is gently placed on an interproximal surface, taking care to avoid any margins. The inlay is gently teased out of the inlay preparation (Fig 9–5). If the inlay resists removal, a loop of dental floss can be placed in a small increment of the composite resin material, and that small amount of composite resin is placed in

the central fossa area of the inlay and light cured. This will act as a handle for engaging an instrument to remove the inlay along the preparation's path of draw.

Oven Tempering. Separator lubricant (Coltene-Whaledent) is painted on all the inlay surfaces. This will act to exclude air and will allow the inlay to completely cure without an air-inhibited layer. The air-inhibited layer is the softest layer of composite resin and should be excluded whenever possible. The inlay is then light cured for an additional 60 seconds (Fig 9–6). The composite resin inlay must now be tempered in an oven. The inlay is heat cured in a DI-500 oven (Coltene-Whaledent; Fig 9–7) or a Cerinate Oven (Den-Mat Corp; Fig 9–8) at 110°C for 7 minutes. The combined light and heat curing ensures complete polymerization of the material, which guarantees an increased hardness and provides potential for increased wear-resistance of the inlay. Polymerization shrinkage in the mouth, which can cause marginal gaps, will also be minimized.

This direct-indirect inlay technique eliminates the need for an impression of the preparation, and the inlay can be finished in a single visit (Fig 9–9).

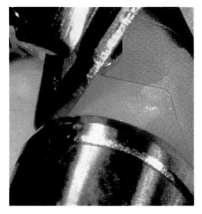

Fig 9–4 All interproximal surfaces have been light cured for 60 seconds. The occlusal surface is then light cured for 60 seconds.

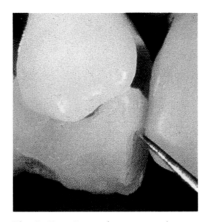

Fig 9–5 Once the composite resin inlay has been light cured, the inlay is gently removed from the cavity preparation.

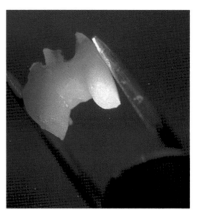

Fig 9–6 After removal from the preparation, the inlay must undergo an additional 60 seconds of light curing prior to oven tempering.

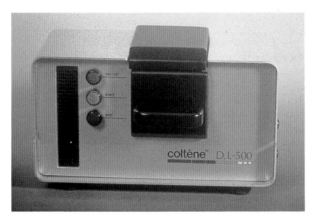

Fig 9–7 DI-500 tempering oven.

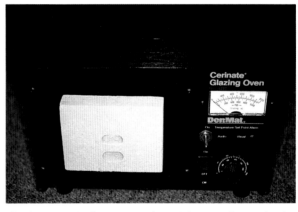

Fig 9–8 A Cerinate oven (Den-Mat Corp) can also be used for heat tempering composite resin inlays.

Fig 9–9 Completed composite resin inlay made from the Brilliant D.I. hybrid resin (Illustration courtesy of Coltene-Whaledent).

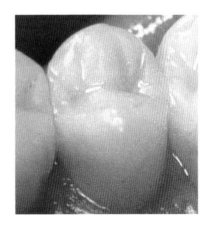

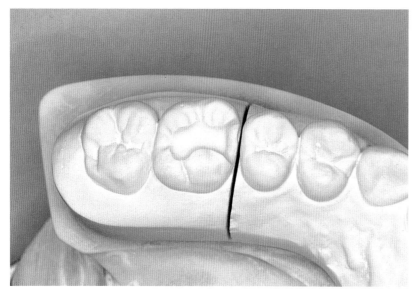

Fig 9–10 After an impression has been made of the inlay preparations, a master cast and dies are made for the fabrication of the composite resin inlay using an indirect technique.

Indirect Technique

The alternative method of composite resin inlay fabrication is to make an impression of the prepared tooth and fabricate the inlay on a die. Examples of these indirect systems are listed in Table 9–1. Recently a versatile composite resin inlay system was introduced. This system (Clearfil CR Inlay, Kuraray) offers a dual-cure composite resin inlay that uses a light for the initiation of polymerization and an inexpensive, compact, heat-curing oven for final hardening of the inlay. This indirect inlay technique can be performed as either a one-visit or two-visit method. The one-visit method involves making an impression with a vinyl polysiloxane material and pouring the impression with a fast-setting die stone such as Snap-Stone (Whip-Mix Corp), which will set within 5 minutes. The inlay is fabricated by the practitioner or staff personnel trained in the technique and should be bonded within approximately 30 minutes. The two-visit method involves sending the impression to a laboratory for fabrication and provides for bonding at a subsequent patient visit. The following description applies to both one-visit and two-visit methods. The difference is in the sequence of the fabrica-tion and whether it takes place in the office or the laboratory. The material used here for demonstration purposes is Clearfil CR Inlay material.

Impression Making. The impression should be made with either a polyether (eg, Polyjel F, LD Caulk/Dentsply International; Impregum F, ESPE-Premier) or a vinyl polysiloxane impression material (eg, Express, 3M; Reprosil, LD Caulk). Either of these materials can be poured in stone immediately and also will remain stable if the impression is sent to a dental laboratory. The impression is then poured up in a die stone for inlay fabrication. For the in-office technique, a fast-setting stone should be used (eg, Snap-Stone, Whip Mix Corp).

Cast Preparation. Once the die stone is set, the cast should be mounted and sectioned in preparation for the inlay fabrication (Fig 9–10). Care should be taken when the cast is sectioned, so that the gingival contacts remain intact; this should be done even at the expense of the adjacent tooth. The impression can be poured a second time if an additional cast is desired to better evaluate the proximal contact area and the path of draw.

Inlay Fabrication. The preparation margins are outlined with a red pencil (Fig 9–11). A separating medium, CR Sep (Kuraray), is applied to the internal surface of the die and also to the surrounding and opposing teeth (Fig 9–12). One or two drops are placed into the cavity preparation and spread over the tooth so that each margin is well coated. The separating medium is then dried with a *gentle* air stream.

The composite resin of the correct shade is dispensed onto a pad. This material is sensitive to light exposure and will cure while it is being worked with, so it is necessary to work quickly. It is advisable to use the material within 5 minutes. The composite resin can be built up in two layers if a shading of dentin and enamel is desired (Fig 9–13). The hybrid composite resin has a high viscosity for ease in sculpting and will hold its shape until light-cured (Fig 9–14). Instruments made specifically for composite resin materials should be used. Proximal and occlusal anatomy should be developed at this stage. Light curing should then be completed; each surface is irradiated for 40 seconds. After light curing, the inlay is removed from the die by pressing on the proximal surface in an occlusal direction (Fig 9–15).

Heat Treatment. The resin inlay is heat treated in an oven for 15 minutes at 100°C in the CRC-100 Curing Oven (Kuraray). This oven can maintain the curing temperature over the curing time for multiple restorations. The unit is very compact and requires little bench-top space (Fig 9–16).

Finishing and Polishing. After heat treatment, the inlay is carved on the die with fine diamonds (Fig 9–17) and mounted abrasive stones (Fig 9–18). The inlay is then polished with composite polishing paste on a buff wheel (Fig 9–19).

Characterization. The inlay is thoroughly cleaned ultrasonically in a water bath. It can then be characterized by applying one of the resin-based colorants provided with the CR Inlay system to the surface of the inlay. This characterizing stain is applied to pits and fissures with a brush. The stain is then light cured for 40 seconds. Stain may also be applied when the composite resin is being layered into the preparation to develop internal characterization. At this stage the inlay is ready for bonding and cementation to the tooth preparation (Fig 9–20).

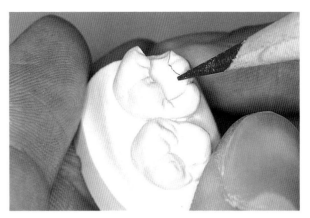

Fig 9–11 A red pencil is used to outline the preparation margins.

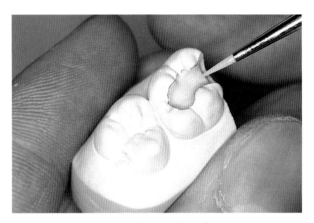

Fig 9–12 The separating medium is painted into the die and on all adjacent cast surfaces.

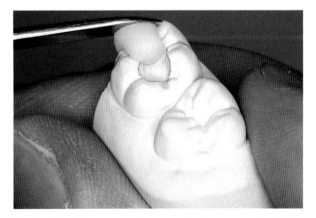

Fig 9–13 The composite resin is placed on the die in two increments.

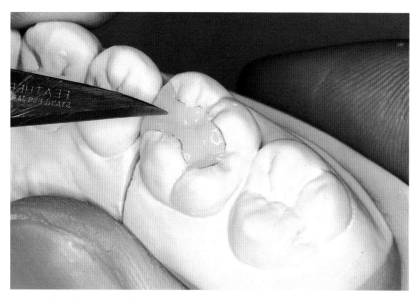

Fig 9–14 The high viscosity of the composite resin allows the occlusal and proximal surfaces to be easily shaped and the composite resin to hold its shape until it is light cured for 40 seconds on each surface.

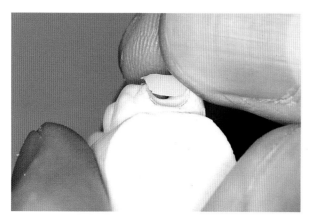

Fig 9–15 The inlay is gently removed from the die after light curing. It is now ready for oven tempering.

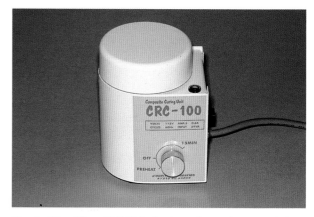

Fig 9–16 The CRC-100 Curing Oven (Kuraray) is a compact heat-tempering oven that will reach a temperature of 100°C and will heat cure the inlay for 15 minutes.

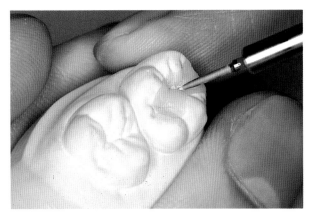

Fig 9–17 The inlay is carved with fine diamonds.

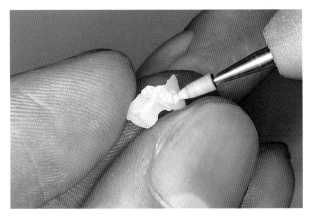

Fig 9–18 The inlay can also be shaped with mounted abrasive stones.

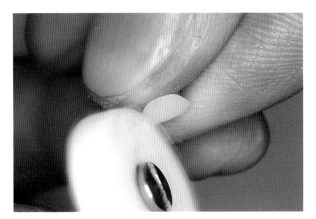

Fig 9–19 The inlay is polished with a buff wheel and composite resin–polishing paste.

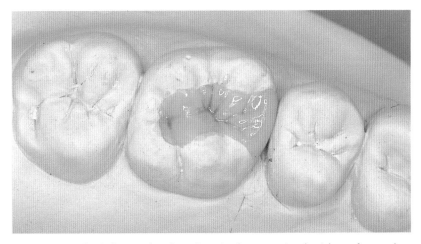

Fig 9–20 The inlay occlusal surface is characterized with surface colorants and then light cured. The inlays are ready for intraoral try-in.

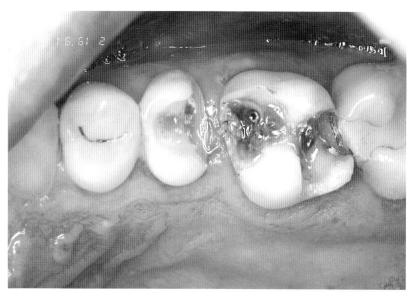

Fig 9–21 The acrylic resin provisional restoration is removed and the preparation is cleaned of all temporary cement.

Removal of the Provisional Restoration

The acrylic resin provisional restoration is carefully removed from the cavity preparation, to avoid damaging the margins of the tooth preparation. A scaler or curet can be used to remove the restoration by placing the end of the instrument on the proximal acrylic resin surface and lifting along the line of draw. Non–eugenol-based temporary cements tend to be softer and less retentive than eugenol-containing cements, so the inlay should be easily dislodged. The preparation is carefully cleaned of any temporary cement (Fig 9–21) and is further cleaned with a prophylaxis brush and a slurry of flour of pumice.

Fit of the Inlay

Before the composite resin inlay is tried into the preparation, the inner surface of the tooth and the restoration are evaluated for irregularities

(Fig 9–22). The inlay should be closely adapted to the working die if the indirect method is being used (Fig 9–23). When the composite resin inlay is tried in, a throat pack of gauze must be placed to protect the patient from aspirating the inlay. The inlay is then gently seated into the preparation. The placement of the contact area and the tightness or looseness of the contact are evaluated by passing unwaxed floss through the proximal contact while an assistant applies pressure on the occlusal surface with a burnisher. If the proximal surface needs to be adjusted, a 5 × 5-mm square piece of Accufilm double-sided articulating film (Parkell) is held in an articulating forceps and placed against the proximal surface of the tooth that is next to the prepared tooth. The inlay is seated and then removed to evaluate the mark on the proximal surface. This area can be adjusted with either a medium Sof-Lex pop-on disk (3M) or an Enhance Sensor disk (LD Caulk/Dentsply International).

Once the inlay is fully seated, it is necessary to verify that the margins of the inlay coincide with the cavosurface margins of the tooth preparation (Fig 9–24). Any excesses can be trimmed with an OS-2 or ET-4 E.T. finishing bur (Brasseler Corp). Interproximal overhangs are trimmed with either an interproximal finishing knife (eg, GKG

38, Hu-Friedy) or a reciprocating handpiece (the Profin, Weissman Technology International) with a safe-sided abrasive point.

For the indirect method, the occlusion should be checked on the die and working cast before the inlay is taken to the mouth. In the direct-indirect method, the occlusion is evaluated prior to the tooth preparation and noted on the diagnostic cast. Any adjustment of opposing teeth necessitated by supereruption or malposition is made prior to tooth preparation. The occlusal form is developed, using the diagnostic casts as a guide. The inlay is replaced on the tooth preparation and the occlusion is checked with Accu-film double-sided articulating film. Care should be taken to have the patient gently tap on the inlay and teeth to avoid fracturing the restoration. If possible, the patient should not be anesthetized during this portion of the procedure. The occlusion is adjusted on the inlay with the Enhance Sensor Disk (LD Caulk/Dentsply International). Care must be taken to verify the occlusal relationships in centric occlusion and in all lateral excursive movements. If occlusal adjustment is necessary, the surface can be recharacterized before final bonding. The final polish of the restoration and refinement of the margins are done after bonding.

Four-Stage Try-in

As with etched porcelain inlays and onlays, each restoration needs to be evaluated for (1) marginal integrity, (2) proximal contact relationship with adjacent teeth, (3) occlusal relationship with the opposing arch, and (4) color. The first three stages have been covered previously in this chapter. The color match of the inlay to the tooth should be within one half of a shade. The shade must blend with that of the existing tooth and adjacent teeth. Occlusal coloration is accomplished during the fabrication; brown and white stains are used to simulate pit and fissure staining and characterization. The color of the cement is selected to be compatible with the shade selected for the composite resin inlay material.

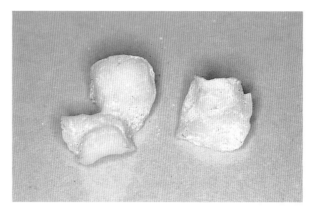

Fig 9–22 The inner aspects of the inlay are inspected for irregularities that might not allow the composite resin restoration to seat on the tooth.

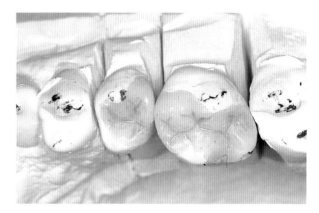

Fig 9–23 Before intraoral try-in, the inlay should be well adapted to the margins of the die.
seat on the tooth.

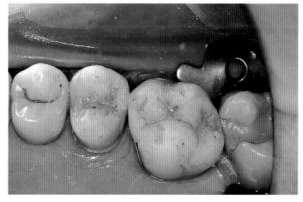

Fig 9–24 The inlay margins are verified while the inlay is fully seated in the tooth preparation.

Placement of the Restoration

Rubber Dam Isolation

Before the inlay is bonded, the rubber dam is placed. Whenever possible, it is advisable to isolate at least two teeth distal to the tooth being restored. This will avoid problems that might occur during inlay seating as a result of clamp jaws that impinge on the gingiva or interproximal area of the tooth. A heavy-weight rubber dam should be used to afford optimal gingival retraction during cementation. The dam can be inverted to seal the area from salivary and hemorrhagic contamination.

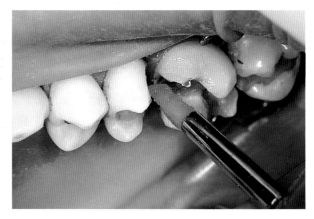

Fig 9–25 The enamel margins of the tooth preparation are etched with a gel etchant for 30 seconds and then rinsed for 20 seconds with a water spray.

Inlay Adjustment

After polymerization, the internal surfaces of the inlay are roughened with an OS-2 diamond (Brasseler Corp) to allow for chemical cross-linking between the cementation agent and the composite resin inlay restoration. The inlay is tried into the preparation and verified for complete seating with the rubber dam in place. With the indirect inlay method, the inlay has already been adjusted on the die. With the direct-indirect method (using the Coltene-Whaledent DI system or the Den-Mat True Vitality system), the gross excesses of the occlusal portion of the inlay must be reduced intraorally on the tooth preparation by using the Brasseler OS-2F diamond without water spray. Care is taken to avoid the preparation margins. The interproximal margins will be finished after cementation. Occlusion will be adjusted after the inlay is bonded to place.

Adhesive Bonding

The tooth is first cleaned with a slurry paste of flour of pumice on a prophylaxis cup. The tooth preparation is then treated with the adhesive. First, the enamel margins are etched with a gel etchant for 30 seconds (Fig 9–25), which is then rinsed from the tooth for 20 seconds with a water spray. The tooth is dried. The dentin and etched enamel are pretreated with an aluminum oxalate dentin conditioner (eg, Tenure, Den-Mat Corp) that is painted into the preparation for 30

seconds. This is then rinsed from the tooth for 15 seconds and the preparation is air dried. The Tenure A and B resin adhesive solutions are mixed together and painted on the etched enamel and dentinal surfaces. This will air dry in 30 seconds. Tenure is selected because of its very low film thickness and because it is a self-curing dentin and enamel bonding adhesive.

The tooth preparation is painted with a very light coating of an unfilled resin (eg, Visar Seal, Den-Mat Corp) that will act as a wetting agent to the Tenure. A dual-cure composite resin cement is selected. The same composite resin cements can be used for porcelain and ceramic inlays as for composite resin inlays. The cement is mixed in accordance with the manufacturer's instructions and applied to the tooth preparation and the internal surface of the inlay (Fig 9–26). The inlay is seated to place with a ball burnisher. A fine, sable-hair paintbrush wetted with unfilled resin is used to gently remove gross excess of the composite resin bonding cement. This will prevent gross excess buildup of the composite resin cement that would need to be finished with rotary instruments after light curing. If the restoration is adjacent to other composite resin restorations, it will be necessary to use a matrix strip interproximally.

The restoration is light cured from all aspects— proximal, facial, lingual, and occlusal—for 60 seconds each (Fig 9–27).

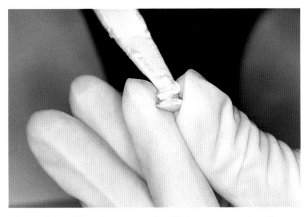

Fig 9–26 The dual-cure (ie, light-cure and self-cure action) cement is mixed and applied to the internal surface of the inlay and the cavity preparation.

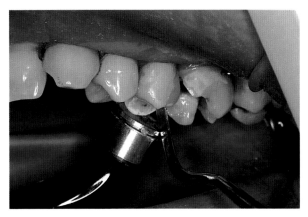

Fig 9–27 The fully seated inlay is light cured on all surfaces for 60 seconds.

Advantages of Composite Resin Inlays

There are several reasons for using composite resin inlays rather than porcelain and directly placed composite resin restorations. Composite resin inlays have been in use in clinical practice, and clinical trials of more than 3 years have shown results equal to or better than those achieved with posterior composite resin restorations. This procedure offers several advantages:

- High esthetics
- Better control of the contact areas
- Excellent marginal adaptation
- Reduced or no laboratory fee if done in the office
- Ready repairability of material intraorally

- Cross-splinting of the compromised tooth and easy removal if replacement becomes necessary
- Compensation for complete polymerization shrinkage by curing the materials outside of the mouth
- Increased composite resin strength because of the heat-curing process

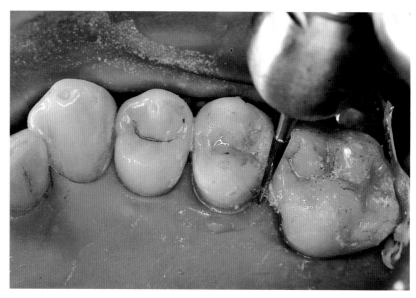

Fig 9–28 After the inlay is light cured, the excess cement is removed from the margins using E.T.-U.F. finishing burs (Brasseler Corp).

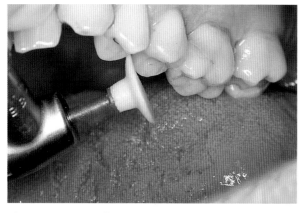

Fig 9–29 An Enhance Sensor Disk is used to create the final margins of the inlay.

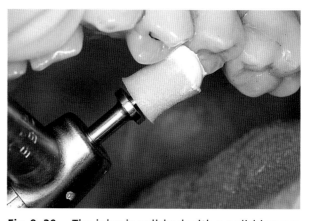

Fig 9–30 The inlay is polished with a polishing cup and composite resin–polishing paste.

Finishing and Polishing

After the composite resin cement has been polymerized, the margins of the restoration are finished with multifluted finishing burs, in sequence, from a nine-bladed bur to a 16-bladed bur to a 30-bladed E.T. finishing bur (Brasseler Corp) (Fig 9–28). If occlusal grooves or fissures need reemphasizing, an OS-3, OS-4, or a 16- or 30-blade carbide can be used. The restoration is then finished and polished with an aluminum oxide polymer disk (Fig 9–29). The final polish is

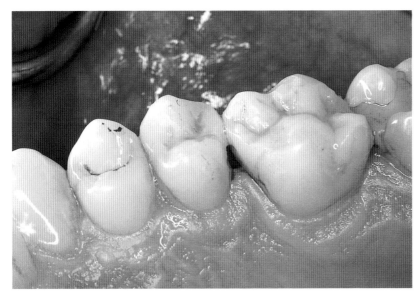

Fig 9–31 Completed CR Inlay restorations.

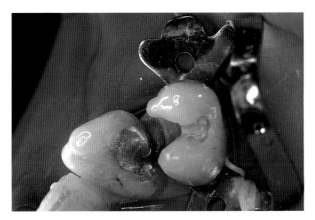

Fig 9–32a Mesio-occlusal inlay preparation on the maxillary first premolar in an esthetic area.

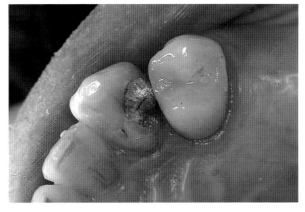

Fig 9–32b Premolar restored with True Vitality composite resin inlay.

accomplished with a composite resin–polishing paste (eg, PrismaGloss, LD Caulk/Dentsply International; Rembrandt Polishing Paste, Den-Mat Corp) on a polishing cup (Fig 9–30). The rubber dam is removed and the inlay's occlusion is verified with Accufilm articulating film in centric occlusion and excursive contacts. If the occlusion is adjusted, then the restoration must be re-polished. Figure 9–31 shows a completed inlay. Figures 9–32a and b show a mesio-occlusal restoration on a maxillary first premolar in an esthetic area.

Expanded Clinical Variations

10

The concept of the etched porcelain, resin-bonded restoration has inspired a plethora of potential uses for this minimally invasive and conservative mode of therapy. Such uses range from porcelain laminate veneers, inlays, crowns, and mini-laminates to anterior etched porcelain fixed partial dentures. Chapters 1 to 7 have covered the more conventional uses in the posterior segment, where this type of bonded restoration restores both functional strength and beauty to the compromised tooth. The more esoteric individual types of etched restorations such as the Class IV etched porcelain restoration and the Class III lingual approach to maintain contact relations and develop guidance, have also been discussed. This chapter expands on these single-tooth restorations and describes the use of two etched porcelain "overlays" to carry a fixed partial denture pontic.

Etched Porcelain Fixed Partial Denture

The need for a conservative approach to congenitally missing or extracted teeth was manifested by the development in the early 1980s of a resin-bonded, etched metal retainer that carried a pontic. This concept has been continually developed to overcome its limitations, and this type of restoration has become an accepted conservative alternative to full-coverage restorations as abutments for a fixed partial denture.

The success of porcelain laminate veneers encouraged some clinicians to expand on their use as retainers for pontics, and in 1986 Ibsen and Strassler published the first article describing an innovative method for a fixed anterior tooth replacement that incorporated etched porcelain veneers. The resin-bonded labial veneers improved the esthetics of the abutment teeth and carried the pontic between them. The concept was further developed to create lingual porce-

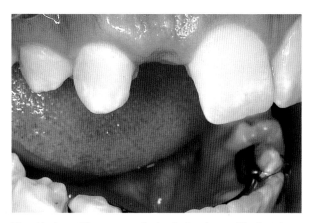

Fig 10–1a The congenital missing lateral incisor is to be replaced with an etched porcelain restoration of two Class III inlay preparations.

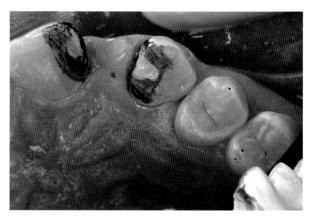

Fig 10–1b Two Class III inlay preparations made from a lingual-buccal approach. (Green stain has been used on the lingual aspects to make the preparation more visible.)

lain veneers, or "wings," to replace preexisting etched metal retainers (ie, Maryland bridges). The porcelain wings did not add strength to the system but merely replaced the missing etched metal retainers for occlusal stability. In those situations where the abutments did not need esthetic modification and no preexisting Maryland bridge was present, a further modification evolved. This was to develop two Class III–type inlay preparations in the abutment teeth with an incisal or lingual path of insertion and use this to carry a pontic (Figs 10–1a to f). These preparations are of necessity always divergent toward the periphery of the tooth to facilitate ease of insertion. They must be designed to provide resistance form to the forces induced during mandibular function and must also act as vertical support in mandibular function.

The ongoing technical progress and development of stronger porcelains reinforced with fibers and other systems (eg, Vita In-Ceram, Vident; Optec, Jeneric/Pentron; Mirage Fibre Reinforced Porcelain, Chameleon Dental Products; Cerinate, Den-Mat Corp) has resulted in ongoing interest in this field. The reason is obvious: these restorations require as conservative a preparation as the conventional etched metal fixed partial dentures, but they are considerably more esthetic. The relatively good success rate of these anterior fixed partial dentures has led investigators to research their uses in posterior situations. The concept has been approached from two distinct aspects: *(1)* the all-ceramic fixed partial denture, and *(2)* metal-reinforced ceramic fixed partial dentures with intracoronal restorations.

When a premolar or first molar is missing, two slot preparations can be created in the adjacent teeth. The potential width and vertical height of each preparation, relative to the tooth, must be maximized to facilitate development of a broad contact area. This broad contact area will then give the connectors the desired strength. If the cross-sectional connector area is sufficiently large, it is possible in specific instances to approach this as an all-porcelain restoration, particularly when the porcelain is of the reinforced type.

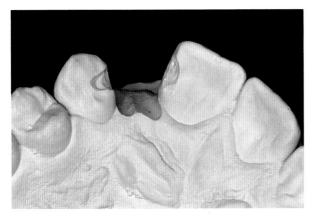

Fig 10–1c Master cast of Class III inlay preparation.

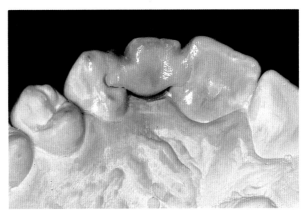

Fig 10–1d Fabricated ceramic restoration in position on the working cast.

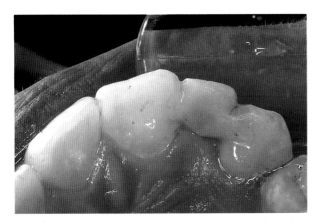

Fig 10–1e Lingual view of the restoration luted in position on the abutments.

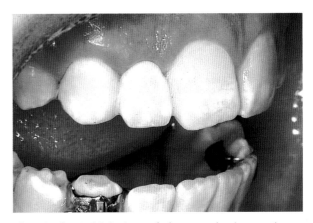

Fig 10–1f Labial view of the prosthesis, postinsertion.

Alternatively, a metal-ceramic bar substructure is used and encased in porcelain. The bar is entirely surrounded by porcelain so that it is the etched surface of the porcelain that is actually bonded to the tooth preparations (Fig 10–2).

The authors have used various modifications of this concept, including a reinforcing or strengthening base metal alloy substructure that rests on the pulpal aspects of the preparation but is covered by porcelain on the occlusal surface and over the pontic (Fig 10–3). If a base metal alloy is used in the cavity base, it can be etched with a solution of hydrofluoric, sulfuric, and nitric acids, while the porcelain against the lateral walls of the preparation is etched with hydrofluoric

acid. If the metal ceramic alloy is one that does not etch effectively, it can still be bonded by sandblasting and treating it with a metal-priming agent before bonding. The prosthesis is bonded to the tooth in the usual manner; a rubber dam is used for complete isolation whenever possible.

The concept can also be used in the anterior section of the mouth by similarly developing two inlay preparations on the adjacent teeth (Figs 10–4a and b). A cast-metal bar is overlaid with ceramic and covers the pontic (Figs 10–4c and d). The final prosthesis is luted in position and creates the illusion of a normal tooth (Fig 10–4e).

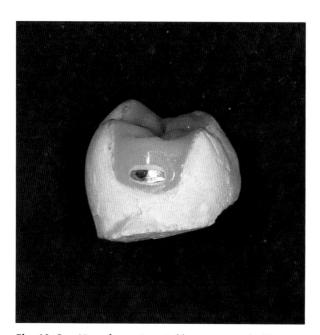

Fig 10–2 Use of a cast-metal bar surrounded by porcelain. The fitting surface of the porcelain is to be etched for luting.

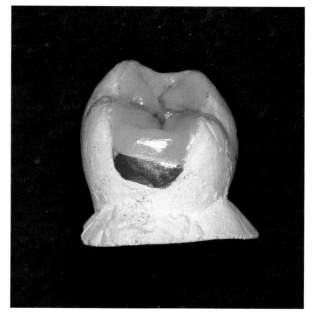

Fig 10–3 Use of an etched cast–base metal alloy on the pulpal aspect of the cavity preparation.

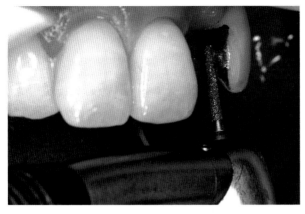

Fig 10–4a A slot inlay preparation is developed for an anterior hybrid metal-ceramic luted fixed partial denture.

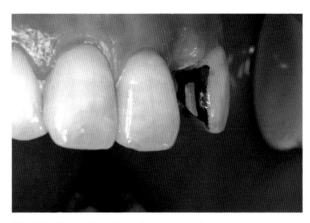

Fig 10–4b Completed preparation on cusp abutment.

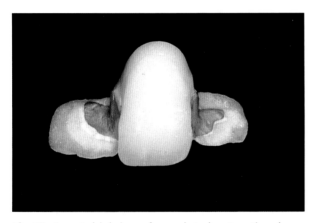

Fig 10–4c Labial view of completed restoration showing reinforcing etched cast-metal bar.

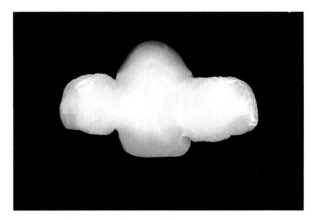

Fig 10–4d Lingual view of restoration showing the metal bar hidden by the porcelain.

Fig 10–4e Completed restoration in position.

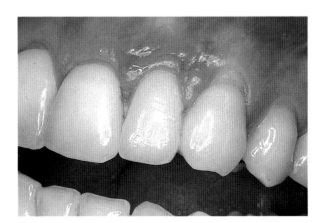

Alternatively, a reinforcing substructure of specialized ceramic, such as In-Ceram (Vident), can be used (Fig 10–5). Some of these core materials cannot be etched, but scanning electron micrographs of the products show that they innately have the type of topographic surface suitable for developing high composite resin bond strengths. Early studies have shown that the bond strength of composite resin to In-Ceram is similar to that of composite resin to etched conventional porcelain.

A useful application for this type of all-ceramic fixed partial denture is when the first molar has been lost and the second molar has tipped and drifted mesially. This change in position invari-ably results in limited contact of the tipped mandibular second molar with the opposing occlusion (Fig 10–6a). The space that now exists between the occlusal surface of the tipped molar and the opposing occlusion (which may not have extruded), provides extra interocclusal space for development of a connector for an all-ceramic fixed partial denture. In these situations an onlay approach is used to increase strength and to redevelop the occlusal harmony (Fig 10–6b). The occlusal surface is roughened to increase adhesion, and all sharp angles are rounded. The buccal and lingual cusps are prepared with a chamfer finish line.

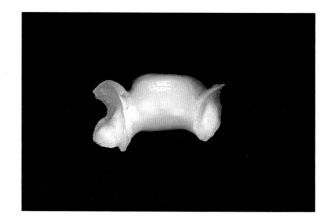

Fig 10–5 Lateral view of an alternative restoration supported by In-Ceram (Vident).

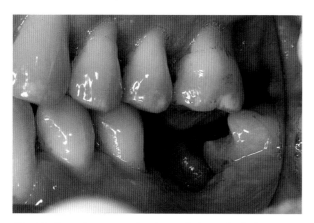

Fig 10–6a Preoperative lateral view of missing mandibular left first molar.

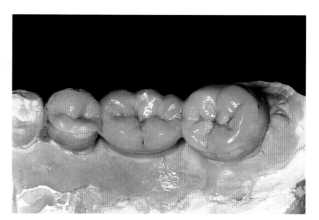

Fig 10–6b Master cast with preparations showing the disto-occlusal inlay on the second premolar and an onlay on the mesially tilted second molar. The vertical discrepancy between the occlusal surfaces allows for a dramatic increase in the amount of porcelain buildup, which increases the strength and restores more function to the side of the arch.

In the mesial abutment, the standard inlay cavity preparation is developed in the distal aspect where there was a preexisting amalgam restoration (Fig 10–7a). The reinforced porcelain is stacked (Fig 10–7b) to articulate with the opposing plane of occlusion in the maxillary arch, which is connected by occlusal reshaping if necessary. Success with this type of all-ceramic fixed partial denture (Fig 10–7c) is predicated on the availability of increased vertical height of the connector space on the mesial aspect of the molar that has been tipped and on the development of optimal occlusal relations with no lateral excursive torquing contacts. Periodontally, the tipped molar should show no evidence of a mesial osseous defect and should be resistant to the inflammatory periodontal process. Otherwise, molar uprighting should be completed and an alternative restoration considered.

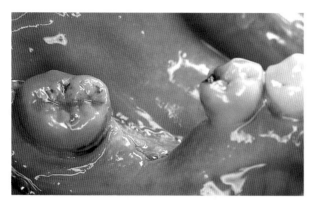

Fig 10–7a Preoperative occlusal view showing tilted molar and an amalgam restoration in the disto-occlusal aspect of the premolar.

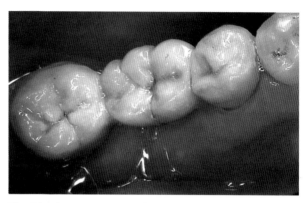

Fig 10–7b Restoration luted in position. It is built up occlusally to the correct plane of occlusion, necessitating an onlay on the molar. This also provides increased strength.

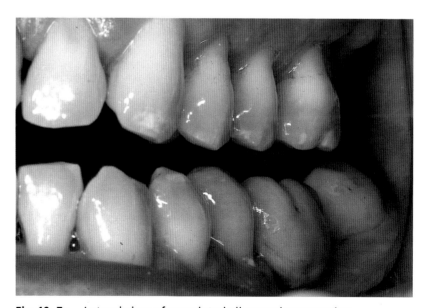

Fig 10–7c Lateral view of completed all-ceramic restoration.

Alteration of Occlusal Arrangement

In clinical practice it sometimes becomes necessary to alter the occlusal arrangement of the teeth. In many of these instances the teeth involved have no restorations and it is undesirable for the clinician to prepare them for the placement of fixed restorations simply to alter the occlusal scheme.

Alternatively, in cases where some form of fixed restoration is already planned in one of the arches, the etched porcelain restoration on the unaltered occlusal surface offers a viable alternative for changing the occlusal arrangement in combination with conventional fixed therapy to retain the fixed partial denture pontics.

Clinical Case (Figs 10–8a to d)

A patient presented with congenitally missing lateral incisors, bilaterally, and a missing maxillary right first premolar. Class III skeletal and edge-to-edge incisal relationships were diagnosed. The patient desired a fixed prosthesis and improvement in overall esthetics.

The prosthesis was designed to incorporate the premolars bilaterally. To develop an increase in the overjet relationship so that the incisal guidance became effective in disarticulating the posterior teeth during excursive movements of the mandible, the vertical dimension was increased. The increase in vertical dimension was evaluated with an occlusal appliance, and this information was transferred to the provisional restoration extending from premolar to premolar. The molars required an increase in vertical dimension to the new plane of occlusion, and to this end occlusal laminate onlays were placed bilaterally. (Orthodontics would have been preferable, but time was a factor.)

In this case the preparation consisted of merely roughening the tooth surface to be covered (thereby improving adhesion) and rounding out any sharp profiles. The buccal, lingual, and interproximal occlusal aspects were prepared with a very mild chamfer so that a definitive finish line was evident for the laboratory technician. The etched porcelain restorations were luted in position at the increased vertical dimension, and the occlusion was adjusted to the terminal arc of closure. A new bite registration was taken, and the anterior fixed conventional prosthesis was fabricated in harmony with these restorations.

It would be prudent to acknowledge that this type of restoration is no panacea. To view it as a conservative, simple method of altering the occlusal arrangement for any given reason would be folly. Before treatment this aggressive is considered (eg, temporomandibular joint syndromes), the occlusion must be tested for its culpability in causing whatever symptoms are involved and effectively indicted. Then before any restorations are bonded in place, the desired occlusal scheme must be worked out in some form of removable appliance to ensure that it will effectively treat the problem over the long term. Many occlusal therapies appear to solve myofunctional pain-dysfunction syndrome only for the short term, before reoccurrence invariably develops. Removable occlusal appliances are more prudent alternatives in most situations.

Conclusion

Potential use of the etched porcelain restoration in its various guises is restricted only by the innovative mind of the clinician or the products' innate strength. As we find ways to increase ceramic strength, so will the conservative modality of therapy increase its range of clinical applications.

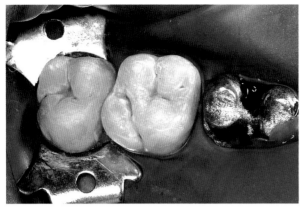

Fig 10–8a Etched preparation of the molars for placement of the occlusal overlays.

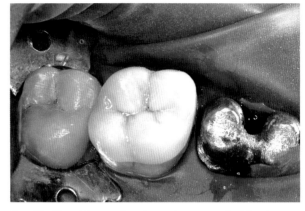

Fig 10–8b The occlusal overlays are tried in the patient's mouth.

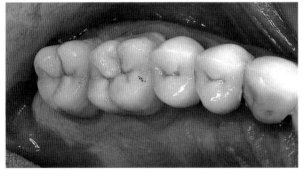

Fig 10–8c The molar occlusal overlays are luted in position adjacent to the metal-ceramic fixed partial denture, which extends anteriorly—all at the increased vertical dimension.

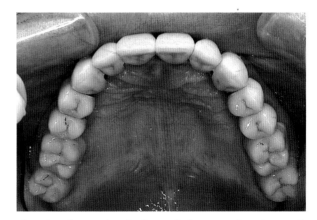

Fig 10–8d Occlusal view of the completed metal-ceramic fixed partial denture and the all-ceramic bonded molar overlays.

Directly Milled Ceramic Inlays and Onlays — CAD/CAM Systems

11

Barry P. Isenberg/David A. Garber

Research and Prototypes

The introduction of computer-aided design/computer-aided manufacture (CAD/CAM) systems to restorative dentistry represents a major technological breakthrough. It is now possible to design and fabricate ceramic restorations at a single appointment, as opposed to the traditional method of making impressions, fabricating a provisional prosthesis, and using a laboratory for development of the restoration. Eliminated are certain errors and inaccuracies that are inherent to the indirect method. Additionally, CAD/CAM–generated restorations save the dentist and patient time, provide an esthetic restoration, and have the potential for extended wear-resistance.

In the past, for intracoronal restorations, the dentist was limited to such materials as amalgam, gold, posterior composite resin, or laboratory-produced resin or ceramic restorations. Although posterior materials have been improved, distinct problems are associated with most of the materials over time. A wear-resistant, esthetic posterior restoration has been difficult to devel-op. Of the materials used, ceramics most closely approximates the properties of enamel (Craig, 1980). If the teeth and ceramic are etched and bonded into the tooth with a composite resin, the resistance to wear and fracture increases; therefore, marginal integrity becomes an important criterion.

Optical scanning and computer generation of restorations were attempted as early as 1971 (Altschuler, 1971/1973). With the continued improvement in the technology, a number of systems are currently being investigated at this time (Duret et al, 1988; Williams, 1987; Rekow, 1987; Brandestini et al, 1985; Duret and Preston, 1991). Additionally, other computer systems for creating dental prostheses are being developed (eg, The Celay System, The Procera System, The Titan System, and several projects from Japan).

It appears that the teams most actively pursuing this technology of CAD/CAM in dentistry are the French group, headed by Dr François Duret, whose system is currently being investigated at the University of Southern California; the Denti-CAD unit at the University of Maryland, led by Dr Dianne Rekow; and the Brandestini/Mörmann unit, working on the Cerec system.

The French system—one of the earliest—was first shown as a prototype in 1983. This system uses lasers to optically scan the image or preparation in the patient's mouth. Multiple images from different angles are obtained with an optical probe. The computer then creates a three-dimensional composite view of the tooth on which the operator can trace the margins of the preparation. With the aid of the computer and adaptations of a theoretical tooth, the external surfaces can be milled with a 3.5-axis-of-rotation machining tool. The system will be capable of milling inlays, onlays, full crowns, and three-unit fixed partial dentures. It is probably the most elaborate, comprehensive, and expensive model being tested. With this system, dentists would most likely have to maintain the probe in the dental office and transmit data to a central laboratory for prosthesis fabrication.

The system that was originally investigated at the University of Minnesota by Dr Dianne Rekow (now at the University of Maryland) originally used a technique described as being "stereophotogrametric." It used a series of black and white photographs to create the tooth contours necessary to rebuild missing parts of the clinical crown. The information was converted to digital form, which was used by a computer to reconstruct the crown. The newest prototype system developed by Rekow, the DentiCAD, uses direct intraoral contact digitization, a form of micropalpation. A tracing probe relays intraoral information of the tooth to the computer. Although this system is still under development and incomplete at this time, it will have the capability of fabricating inlays, onlays, and complete crowns from resins, ceramics, and metals.

The third system, the Cerec system, developed in Zürich, Switzerland, has been available in Europe for 8 years and is currently being marketed in the United States, Canada, Japan, Mexico, South Africa, and South America by the Siemens Corporation. It is the system that will be discussed here, as it is one that is commercially available and practical for the dental office at this time. This CAD/CAM unit, which will fabricate inlays, onlays, ¾ crowns, ⅞ crowns, and veneers, will allow the clinician to restore the tooth with an indirect, permanent restoration in one appointment. This is done without the use of an impression or the assistance of a laboratory technician. The compact, mobile unit can be seen in Fig 11–1. It consists of three basic components: a small camera (Fig 11–2), a computer with screen (Fig 11–3), and a three-axis-of-rotation milling machine (Fig 11–4). A new version of the milling motor has been introduced. It uses an electric motor ("E" version) to drive the milling wheel instead of the water-pressure-driven "hydro" version. This provides a smoother cutting of the ceramic, hence a better fitting restoration.

A flow diagram describing the Cerec system is given in Fig 11–5. The scan head of the camera emits infrared light through the lens onto the surface of the prepared tooth. The light is reflected back into the scanning head and onto a photoreceptor, which is conveyed to the computer. The intensity of the reflected light is recorded as values that give vertical dimension to the depth of the cavity preparation. The recorded data are then transferred from the memory of the computer to the small milling machine, which fabricates the restoration.

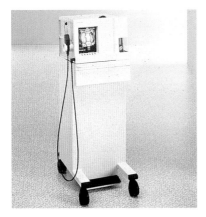

Fig 11–1 The compact, mobile Cerec unit, which incorporates a camera, the computer components and screen, and a three-access-of-rotation milling machine (Pelton & Crane, a division of Siemens).

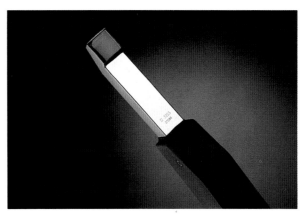

Fig 11–2 The camera used to capture the optical impression.

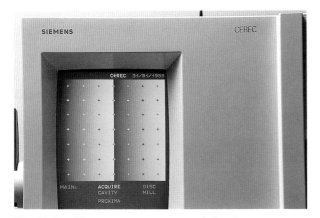

Fig 11–3 The computer screen of the Cerec system.

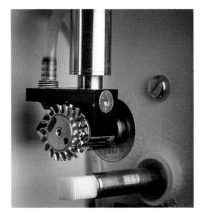

Fig 11–4 The three-access-of-rotation milling machine used to fabricate the restoration.

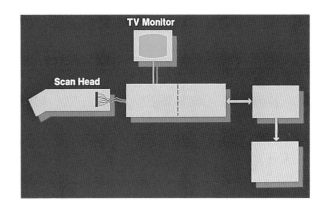

Fig 11–5 A flow diagram of the process of manufacturing a restoration using the Cerec system.

Clinical Procedure for the Cerec System

Preparation Design

There are certain prerequisites for the preparation design for a Cerec restoration. The conventional inlay design must be modified to best use the capabilities of the milling device. The computer *cannot accurately read bevels, convexities, steps, or undefined angles*; it is therefore imperative that *the prepared walls be as straight as possible*. The ideal occlusal wall can be vertical, slightly convergent, or slightly divergent to the occlusal cavosurface (Fig 11–6). In general, a slightly *convergent* wall lends itself to a sharper image on the screen; hence it is easier for the computer to read. If an undercut portion is generated during the preparation procedure, it will be blocked out during imaging and become filled in with the luting composite resin. The occlusal cavosurface should have a smooth, flowing outline.

Proximal walls with a slight occlusal *divergence* and a flare into the proximal through the contact allow the operator to place the boundaries of the restoration as close as possible to the gingival cavosurface angle.

Floors and walls that are relatively flat give the computer an image that is more discernible and allow a much more intimate fit, especially at the margin. In instances of very deep lesions with close proximity to the pulp, a hard-setting or light-cured calcium hydroxide base should be placed. To level the pulpal floor and cavity walls and provide additional pulpal protection, a glass-ionomer base should be placed over the remaining dentin. Irregular surfaces make it more difficult for the milling machine to accurately mill the ceramic material.

The Optical Impression

The surface of the prepared tooth often lacks sufficient reflectivity, or it may have facets that give an uneven glare to the computer screen. It is therefore necessary to coat the preparation with a special powder that has the proper light-reflective ability (Fig 11–7). A rubber dam should be used to obtain complete tissue and moisture

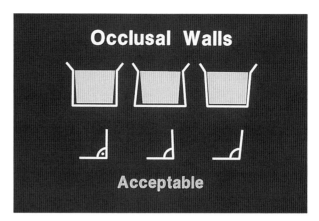

Fig 11–6   Desirable configurations of the cavity wall.

isolation, because oral fluids may contaminate the powder, and the humidity of the oral cavity will tend to fog the camera and give a less-than-clear image.

A hand-held camera is placed over the prepared, powder-coated cavity to obtain a fixed image on the computer screen. The camera is adjusted until a clear image and all aspects of the cavity can be seen. It is essential to position the camera over the long axis so that the computer can read all internal walls and cavosurfaces equally. At this point the operator, by releasing the foot pedal, "freeze frames" the preparation on the screen. The focal length of the camera lens is 10 mm; any depth greater than 10 mm will not focus properly and an ill-fitting restoration subsequently will be generated.

Computer-Generated Restoration Design

The restoration is designed from the image shown on the computer screen by using a series of icons or symbols. The operator can electronically design the restoration by moving a cursor along the limits of the preparation, thereby defining its boundaries. The internal limits are created, as are the walls and cavosurface margins. Thus, the gingival floors, axial walls, cavosurface margins, proximal contours (contacts), and marginal ridges are established (Fig 11–8). The procedure can be stopped at any time and edited to override the computer and allow the operator to correct the electronically generated features. Once the res-

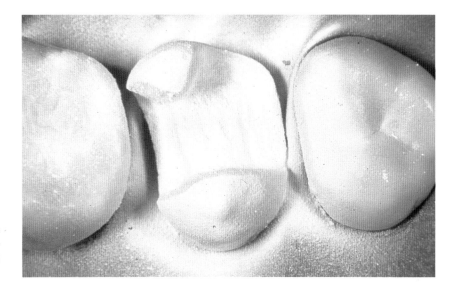

Fig 11–7 The cavity preparation is coated with a light-reflective powder to facilitate optical impression making.

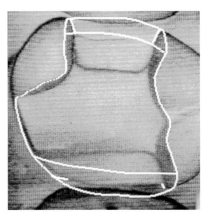

Fig 11–8 The restoration is electronically determined with a cursor to delineate the outline form and the internal limits.

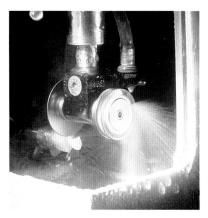

Fig 11–9 The ceramic block is inserted into the milling machine, which is activated to grind out the restoration.

toration has been designed, the computer develops an on-screen, three-dimensional model or image of the inlay, onlay, or veneer. All of the information generated is stored automatically on a programmed floppy disk. Up to three images may be stored on each disk. The design phase usually takes from 2 to 8 minutes. This is even possible when designing multiple cusp replacements or veneers.

Milling Procedure

After all the data have been supplied, the com-

puter selects the size of ceramic block to be used in the milling process. There is a wide range of shades and sizes of both porcelain (Vita, Vident Co) and castable ceramic (Dicor, Dentsply International). These blocks are factory-fabricated and thus are more homogeneous and less porous than material that is traditionally made in the dental laboratory. The material is mounted on a metal stub, which allows it to be inserted into the milling unit. Once the material is inserted, the small window is closed and the milling device is activated (Fig 11–9). The milling is accomplished by a three-axis-of-rotation cutting machine, which mills 25-μm slices. A diamond wheel is driven by the electric motor, which generally takes 4 to 7 minutes to complete the procedure. The milling allows for occlusal contours of the cuspal inclines, marginal ridges, and proximal contours. It does not provide for internal and secondary occlusal anatomy. This is developed by the operator intraorally after the inlay has been cemented.

Clinical Placement

Because breakdown primarily occurs at the tooth-restoration interface, the interfacial gap and luting agent play an important role in longevity of the restoration. The gap should be kept under 100 μm, particularly on the occlusal surface (Leinfelder et al, 1989). Wear, staining, secondary caries, and possibly marginal fracture could be expected if the gap were excessive. Recent studies (Isenberg et al, 1990, 1992) indicate that if the gap is small, the wear is minimal. Once fit has been assessed, the restoration can be cemented in place.

Cementation involves etching the tooth with a 37% solution of phosphoric acid for 20 seconds. The tooth is then washed and dried and a bonding agent is applied. The ceramic restoration is etched on its undersurface, *outside the mouth.*

Currently the two materials of choice are the Dicor ceramic material and Vita porcelain. The Dicor is etched with ammonium bifluoride, and the Vita is etched with a buffered hydrofluoric acid gel. With either material, a silane coupling agent must be applied to the undersurface for better retention to the composite resin luting agent.

The Dicor material at this time appears to more closely resemble the surface hardness of enamel; consequently the potential for abrasion of the tooth enamel by the antagonist is minimized. Vita recently introduced a new generation of porcelain, Vita Mark II, which has a much smaller particle size. It is currently being evaluated for its wear-resistance and milling characteristics.

At this point a dual-cure microfill composite resin luting agent is used to bond the inlay, onlay, or veneer. Research has shown that the microfill-particle composite resin wears two to three times better than a hybrid composite resin. Once photocuring has been achieved, the occlusal anatomy can be created. This is accomplished intraorally with fine-particle diamonds. The Brasseler system of diamonds is excellent to make the final finishing and polishing using diamonds, 12- and 30-bladed carbide burs, rubber points, and diamond paste.

Advantages of the Cerec System

Ceramic-bonded restorations offer a wide range of advantages over conventional restorative materials. The Cerec CAD/CAM system offers several distinct advantages:

- Single appointment
- No impression
- Bonded restoration for strength
- Reduced marginal gap
- Wear hardness similar to enamel
- Less fracture of the inlay, because it is milled from a solid, homogeneous block
- Excellent polishing characteristics

- Improved esthetics
- Less reduction of tooth structure, hence better periodontal health
- Bonded restorations enhance tooth strength
- Preparation, fabrication, cementation, and polishing normally accomplished in 1 to 1½ hours

---

The Celay System

An innovative system, the Celay technique (developed by Dr Stefan I. Eidenbenz at the University of Zürich), is a variation on the direct-indirect restoration concept but without the need for a laboratory technician. An inlay or onlay preparation is made for the compromised tooth, but, instead of a conventional impression, a direct process is used. A moldable, precision imprint material is modeled directly inside the mouth in the cavity preparation, where it is adjusted for occlusion, contact relations, and marginal integrity. The material then undergoes a light-hardening or curing process before it is removed from the tooth to serve as a prototype model to be copied and reproduced in ceramic on a unique milling system (Fig 11–10) developed by Claude Nowak of Microna Technologie AG, Spreitenbach, Germany.

The milling center has two distinct aspects. In one half the model to be copied is centered in a holder (Fig 11–11), where it is manually scanned (Fig 11–12). A second part of the milling machine contains a rotary turbine (Fig 11–13) with various cutting tools (Fig 11–14). The directly formed pattern in the vise is manually scanned with a sensor. This sensor is directly connected to the milling aspect. Any form scanned is thus simultaneously reproduced in all three dimensions in a block of ceramic by the rotary turbine. The gross form is developed with a diamond disk (Fig 11–15) and refined with a diamond point (Fig 11–16). The ceramic blocks to be milled into restorations are available in various colors and sizes. An appropriately sized block is selected and inserted in the holder of the milling center.

The system can also be used as a purely indirect process, in which an impression is made and a die developed in the laboratory. The composite resin imprint prototype material is precisely formed in the die to represent the desired restoration. The composite resin prototype inlay is then placed in the left side of the milling unit in a bipoint metallic vise (see Fig 11–12). The surface of the prototype is then similarly scanned manually (see Fig 11–13) and reproduced in ceramic on the milling unit, which carves out an exact replica of the plastic prototype in ceramic. The occlusal scheme developed inside the mouth is reproduced identically (Fig 11–17), so that after com-

pletion of the milling process, the inlay is ready to be inserted into the mouth with, at best, minor corrections (Fig 11–18). Additional characterization or colorization of the inlay, if required, can be accomplished in the laboratory by refiring the inlay prior to final finishing (Fig 11–19).

The fit of the restoration has a tolerance of less than 50 μm.

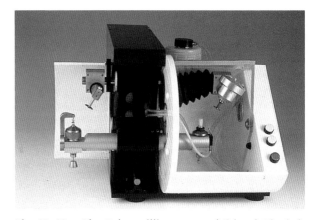

Fig 11–10 The Celay milling system (Vident). The left side has a scanning sensor, which is manually guided over the plastic prototype. The right side of the machine then simultaneously carves out of ceramic a replica of the left side, resulting in marginal integrity of less than 50 μm. (Figures 11–10 through 11–19 courtesy of Microna Technologie AG.)

Advantages of the Celay System

- A precisely fitting ceramic restoration can be developed in one patient session.
- A ceramic restoration can be developed without the need for a laboratory technician.
- The restoration is developed in factory-fired high-grade porcelain.
- The processing time required is very short. A small inlay can be milled in 3 minutes, a mesio-occlusodistal inlay in less than 8 minutes, and a complete onlay in 12 to 13 minutes.

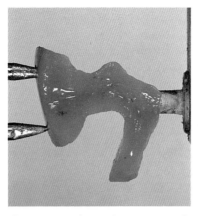

Fig 11–11 The resin prototype is held in position in the jig on the left side of the machine and scanned manually.

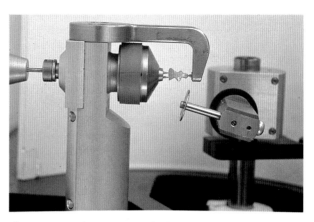

Fig 11–12 The ceramic block is inserted into the milling machine.

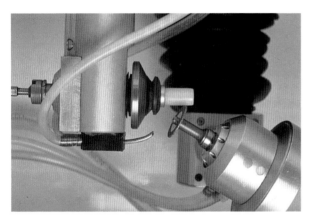

Fig 11–13 The milling machine replicates the resin prototype by using a diamond disk.

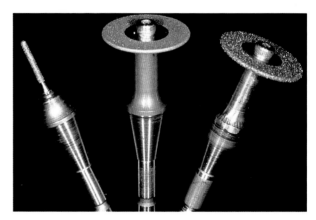

Fig 11–14 The three types of diamond-coated milling instruments in the Celay system.

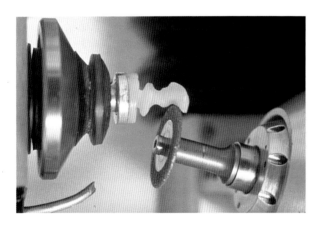

Fig 11–15 The gross form is developed with a diamond disk.

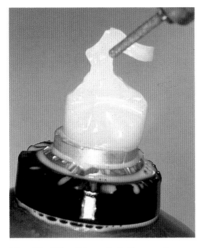

Fig 11–16 Fine details, such as a central fossa and secondary anatomy, are developed with a fine diamond point on the milling machine.

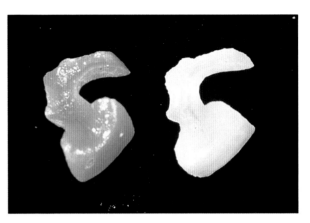

Fig 11–17 A mesio-occlusal buccal acrylic resin prototype restoration *(left)* and its replica in porcelain *(right)*.

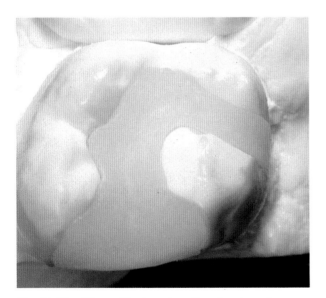

Fig 11–18 The milled restoration is placed on an indirect cast.

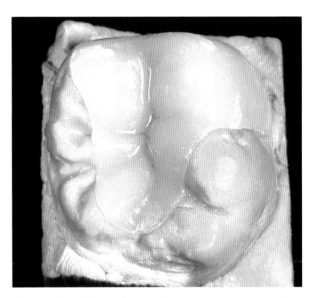

Fig 11–19 A typical completed restoration is tried on an indirect cast to show marginal integrity, occlusal carvings, staining, and final tooth form.

References

Adair PJ, Bell B, Pameijer CH. Casting technique of machinable glass ceramics. *J Dent Res* 1980;59:475 (abstr no. 883).

Adair PJ, Grossman DG. The castable ceramic crown. *Int J Periodont Rest Dent* 1984;2:33–45.

Adair PJ, Hoekstra KE. Fit of castable ceramic. *J Dent Res* 1982;61:345 (abstr no. 1500).

Adair PJ, Sackett BP, Cammarato VT. Preliminary clinical evaluation of cast ceramic full crown restorations. *J Dent Res* 1982;61:292 (abstr no. 1024).

Altschuler BR. Holodontography: An Introduction to Dental Laser Holography. SAM-TR-73-4 Report, No. AD758191. Brooks AFB, Texas, USAF, School of Aerospace Medical Div(AFSC) 1971/1973;78:285.

Bailey LF, Bennett RJ. Dicor surface treatments for enhanced bonding. *J Dent Res* 1988;67:925 (abstr no. 931).

Bennett RJ, Bailey LF. Bonding to Dicor laminate veneers. *J Dent Res* 1986;65:314 (abstr no. 1309).

Biederman JD. Direct composite resin inlay. *J Prosthet Dent* 1989:62:249–253.

Black GC. The physical properties of the silver-tin amalgams. *Dent Cosmos* 1896;38:965.

Blackman R, Barghi N, Duke E. Influence of ceramic thickness on resin curing time. *J Dent Res* 1988:67:305 (abstr no. 1537).

Bleiholder RF, Pijawka JP, Jurecic A. Filler/binder interaction in dental composites. *J Dent Res* 1974;53:151 (abstr no. 387).

Bowen RL. Dental filling material comprising vinyl silane treated fused silica and a binder consisting of a reaction product of bisphenol and glycidyl, methacrylate [US patent 3,066,112], 1962.

Bowen RL. Compatibility of various materials with oral tissues. I: The components in composite restorations. *J Dent Res* 1979;58:1493–1506.

Brandestini M, Mörmann W, Lutz F, Krejci I. Computer machined ceramic inlays: in vitro marginal adaptation. *J Dent Res* 1985;64:208 (abstr no. 305).

Brännström M, Neyborg H. The presence of bacteria in cavities filled with silicate cement composite resin materials. *Swed Dent J* 1971;64:149–153.

Brännström M, Torstenson B, Nordenvall KJ. The initial gap around large composite restorations in vitro: the effect of etching enamel walls. *J Dent Res* 1984;63:681–684.

Buonocore MG. A simple method of increasing the adhesion of acrylic filling materials to enamel surfaces. *J Dent Res* 1955;34:849–853.

Buonocore MG. Principles of adhesive retention and adhesive restorative materials. *J Am Dent Assoc* 1963;67:382–391.

Calamia JR, Calamia S, Lemier J, Hamburg M, Scherer W, Nyucd N. Clinical evaluation of etched porcelain laminate veneers: results at 6 months–3 years. *J Dent Res* 1987;66:245 (abstr no. 1110).

Calamia JR, Simonsen RJ. Effect of coupling agents on bond strength of etched porcelain. *J Dent Res* 1984;63:162 (abstr no. 79).

Calamia J, Vaidynathan J, Calamia S, Hamburg M. Shear bond strength between acid-etched Dicor and composite resin. *J Dent Res* 1986;65:828 (abstr no. 925).

Candio SJ. The direct resin inlay: clinical protocol. *Oral Health* 1990;80(8):9–15.

Cavel WT, Kelsey WP, Barkmeier WW, Blankenau RJ. A pilot study of the clinical evaluation of castable ceramic inlays and a dual-cure resin cement. *Quintessence Int* 1988;19:257–262.

Chan DCN, Jensen ME, Shet J, Sigler T. Shear bond strengths of etched porcelain bonded with resin to enamel. *J Dent Res* 1987;66:245 (abstr no. 1109).

Ciucchi B, Bouillaguet S, Holz J. Proximal adaptation and marginal seal of posterior composite resin restorations placed with direct and indirect techniques. *Quintessence Int* 1990;21:663–669.

Craig RG. *Restorative Dental Materials*, ed 7. St Louis; CV Mosby Co, 1980.

Duret F, Blouin JL, Duret B. CAD/CAM in dentistry. *J Am Dent Assoc* 1988;117:715–720.

Duret F, Preston JD. CAD/CAM imaging in dentistry. *Current Opinion Den* 1991;1:150–154.

Eden GT, Kacicz JM. Dicor crown strength improvement due to bonding. *J Dent Res* 1987;66:207 (abstr no. 801).

Fuzzi M, Luthy H, Wohlwend A, DiFebo G, Carnevale G, Caldari R. Marginal fit of three different porcelain onlays bonded to tooth: an in vitro study. *Int J Periodont Rest Dent* 1991;11:303–315.

Gerbo LR, Leinfelder KF, Mueninghoff LA, Russell C. Use of optical standards for determining wear of posterior composite resins. *J Esthet Dent* 1990;2:148–152.

Gettleman L. Status report on low-gold content alloys for fixed prostheses. *J Am Dent Assoc* 1980;100:237.

Goldstein R. Finishing of composites and laminates. *Dent Clin North Am* 1989;33:305–318.

Gray AW. Volume changes accompany solution, chemical combination and crystallization in amalgam. *Inst Metals J* 1923;29:139.

Grossman DG. Machinable glass-ceramics based on tetrasilic mica *J Am Ceram Soc* 1972;55:446–449.

Hinoura K, Moore BK, Swartz ML, Phillips RW. Tensile bond strength between glass-ionomer cement and composite resin. *J Dent Res* 1986;65:344 (abstr no. 1576).

Hsu CS, Stangel I, Nathanson D. Shear bond strength of resin to etched porcelain. *J Dent Res* 1985;64:296 (abstr no. 1095).

Ibsen RL, Strassler HE. An innovative method for fixed anterior tooth replacement utilizing porcelain veneers. *Quintessence Int* 1986;17:455–459.

Isenberg BP, Essig ME, Leinfelder KF, Mueninghoff LA. Clinical evaluation of CEREC CAD-CAM restorations *J Dent Res* 1990;69:1597 (abstr no. 1597).

Isenberg BP, Essig ME, Leinfelder KF. Three year clinical evaluation of CAD/CAM restorations. *J Esthet Dent* 1992;4:234–238.

Lacy AM, Zhang K, Koh A, Wiltshire WA, Watanabe L. Marginal microleakage around Class II resin and Dicor inlays. *J Dent Res* 1988;67:196 (abstr no. 699).

Landy NA, Simonsen RJ. Cusp fracture strength in Class II composite resin restorations. *J Dent Res* 1984;63:175 (abstr no. 40).

Leinfelder KF, Isenberg BP, Essig ME. A new method for generating ceramic restorations: a CAD-CAM system. *J Am Dent Assoc* 1989;118:703–707.

Leinfelder KF, Price WG, Gurley WH. Low gold alloys: a laboratory and clinician evaluation. *Quint Dent Technol* 1981;5:483.

Leinfelder KF, Roberson TM. Clinical evaluation of posterior composite resins. *Gen Dent* 1983;31:276–281.

Leinfelder KF, Taylor DF. Current status of composite resins. *NC Dent J* 1978;61:17–18.

Litkowski LJ. A review of five dentin-bonding systems. *Esthetic Dent Update* 1990;1(4):58–61.

Ludwig KL. Studies on the ultimate strength of all-ceramic crowns. *Dent Labor* 1991;39:647–651.

Lutz R, Krejci I, Luescher B, Oldenburg TR. Improved proximal margin adaptation of Class II composite resin restorations by use of light-reflecting wedges. *Quintessence Int* 1986;17:659–664.

McInnes-Ledoux PM, Ledoux WR, Weinberg R, Rappold A. Luting castable ceramic restorations—a bond strength study. *J Dent Res* 1987;66:207 (abstr no. 802).

McLean JW, Powis DR, Prosser HJ, Wilson AD. The use of glass-ionomer cements in bonding composite resins to dentine. *Br Dent J* 1985;158:410–414.

Millstein PL, Nathanson D. Effect of eugenol and eugenol cements on cured composite resin. *J Prosthet Dent* 1983;50:211–215.

Millstein PL, Nathanson D. Effects of temporary cementation of permanent cement retention to composite resin cores. *J Prosthet Dent* 1992;67:856–859.

Morin D, DeLong R, Douglas WH. Cusp reinforcement by the acid-etch technique. *J Dent Res* 1984;63:1075–1078.

Nathanson D, Hassan F. Effect of etched porcelain thickness on resin-porcelain bond strength. *J Dent Res* 1987;66:245 (abstr no. 1107).

Peutzfeldt A, Asmussen E. A comparison of accuracy in seating and gap formation for three inlay/onlay techniques. *Oper Dent* 1990;15:129–135.

Rappold A, McInnes-Ledoux P, Zink J, Crowe RA, Weinberg R. Intracoronal cast ceramic restorations—an in vitro investigation of fit. *J Dent Res* 1987;67:134 (abstr no. 218).

Redford DA, Jensen ME. Cuspal flexure, strength, microleakage. *J Dent Res* 1986;65:344 (abstr no. 1573).

Rekow D. Computer-aided design and manufacturing in dentistry: a review of the state of the art. *J Prosthet Dent* 1987;58:512–516.

Robinson PB, Moore BK, Swartz ML. Comparison of microleakage in direct and indirect composite resin restorations in vitro. *Oper Dent* 1987;12:113–116.

Roulet J-F. The problems associated with substituting composite resins for amalgam: a status report on posterior composites. *J Dent* 1988;16:101–113.

Roulet J-F, Herder S. *Bonded Ceramic Inlays*. Chicago, Quintessence Publishing Co, 1991, p 90.

Scherer W, Caliskan F, Kain J, Moss S, Vijayaraghavan T. Comparison of microleakage between direct placement composites and direct composite inlays. *Gen Dent* 1990;38:209–211.

Shortall AC, Baylis RL, Baylis MA, Grundy JR. Marginal seal comparisons between resin-bonded Class II porcelain inlays, posterior composite restorations and direct composite resin inlays. *Int J Prosthodont* 1989;2:217–223.

Stephens EB, Button GL, Gunsolley JC. Knoop microhardness comparison: heat-tempered vs light-cured composite resin. *J Dent Res* 1990;69:310 (abstr no. 1615).

Strassler HE, Nathanson D. The new generation of dentin bonding agents. *Alpha Omegan* 1988;81(12):28–32.

Takeshige F, Kawai K, Torii M, Tsuchitani Y. Effect of heating on physical properties of composite resin. *J Dent Res* 1990; 69:310 (abstr no. 1609).

Wendt SL Jr. The effect of heat used as a secondary cure upon the physical properties of three composite resins. II. Wear, hardness, and color stability. *Quintessence Int* 1987;18: 351–356.

Wendt SL, Leinfelder KF. The clinical evaluation of heat-treated composite resin inlays. *J Am Dent Assoc* 1990; 120:177–181.

Williams AG. The Switzerland and Minnesota developments in CAD/CAM. *J Dent Pract Adm* 1987;4:50–54.

Wilson AD, McLean JW. *Glass-Ionomer Cement*. Chicago, Quintessence Publishing Co, 1988.

Index

history of, 13–21
provisional, 57–65
  direct method, 61
  direct-indirect method, 57
  for composite resin inlays,
    119
  indirect method, 62
  removal, 86, 128
  removal of old, 26, 40
  seating of, 94
  surface contaminants, 86
Denture, partial, fixed, etched
  porcelain, 133
Dies, refractory, 71, 76

F

Fillers, particle size, 18–19

G

Glass-ionomers, 45, 54
Gold alloys
  advantages, 17
  composition, 17
  deformation (bending), 33
  disadvantages, 17
  elasticity, 33
  longevity, 17
  low-gold, 17
  properties of, 18

I

Impressions, 57–65
  fabrication, 65
  preoperative alginate, 57
  techniques for, 64
  tissue management, 64
  vacuform shell, 57, 61
Inlays
  composite resin, 21, 117–131
    adjustment, 128
    advantages, 21, 129
    bonding, 128
    cast preparation, 122
    characterization, 123
    design principles, 118
    direct-indirect method, 119

disadvantages, 21
fabrication, 119, 123, 125
finishing, 123, 130
fit, 126
four-stage try-in, 127
heat-cured, 21
heat treatment, 123
impressions for, 122
indirect method, 122
lubrication, 119
material placement, 119
oven tempering, 120
placement, 128
polishing, 123, 130
provisionalization, 119
removal from investment,
  120, 126
treatment planning, 117
directly milled ceramic,
  143–151
etched porcelain, 23–31
  abrasion resistance, 29
  advantages, 29
  Class III, 50
  Class IV, 52
  color of, 28–29, 31
  contraindications, 24
  design parameters, 27, 37
  disadvantages, 29
  evaluation of, 83
  features, 23–31
  indications, 24
  loading, 34
  microleakage, 23, 29
  placement procedures,
    91–103
  principles of use, 33–38
  radiodensity, 29, 31
  temporary cements for, 37
  tooth preparation, 26–28,
    30, 37, 45, 51–52
vs onlays, 46
Investments
  refractory techniques, 67, 72
  restoration release from, 79,
    120

L

Laboratory procedures, 67–80

Luting, preparation for, 90, 94
Luting agents, composite resin,
  90, 94

M

Matrix, 57, 61, 119

O

Occlusion, altered
  arrangement, 140
Onlays
  composite resin, 21
    advantages, 21
    disadvantages, 21
    heat-cured, 21
  directly milled ceramic,
    145–151
  etched porcelain, 23–31
    abrasion resistance, 29
    advantages, 29
    approximal, 47
    Class II, 44
    color of, 28–29, 31
    contraindications, 24
    cuspal preparation, 47
    design parameters, 27, 37
    disadvantages, 29
    evaluation of, 83
    features, 23–31
    indications, 24
    loading, 34
    microleakage, 23, 29
    placement procedures,
      91–103
    principles of use, 33–38
    radiodensity, 29, 31
    slot preparation, 47
    temporary cements for, 37
    tooth preparation, 26–28,
      30, 37, 45
  vs inlays, 46

P

Porcelain
  anti-"crack propagation"
  force, 35